BARRON'S PARENTING KEYS

KEYS TO BREAST FEEDING

William Sears, M.D.

Pediatrician
Assistant Clinical Professor of
Pediatrics at the University of
Southern California

Martha Sears, R.N.

International Board of
Certified Lactation Consultants

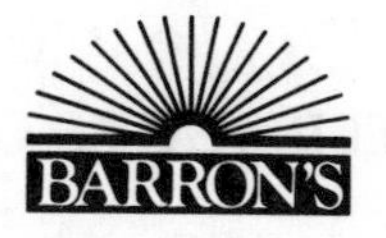

New York • London • Toronto • Sydney

Cover photo by Scott Barrow, Inc., Cold Spring, NY

Illustrations by Marika Hahn

All inquiries should be addressed to:
Barron's Educational Series, Inc.
250 Wireless Boulevard
Hauppauge, New York 11788

Library of Congress Catalog Card No. 90-20688

International Standard Book No. 0-8120-4540-8

Library of Congress Cataloging in Publication Data
Sears, William, M.D.
Keys to successful breastfeeding / by William Sears and Martha Sears.
p. cm.
Includes index.
ISBN 0-8120-4540-8
1. Breastfeeding. I. Sears, Martha. II. Title.
RJ216.S42 1991
649'.33—dc20 90-20688
CIP

PRINTED IN THE UNITED STATES OF AMERICA
1234 5500 987654321

CONTENTS

INTRODUCTION

Welcome to motherhood. Because you have chosen to breastfeed your baby, you have embarked on a journey unique to lactating mothers. By providing the milk from your breast you are guaranteeing the best nourishment and best nurturing for your baby. You are tapping into a formula for mothering and feeding as old as time itself, tested and true. The only thing left to do now is to get started and to enjoy what nature has intended to be your baby's rightful heritage.

The material in this book is based upon our experience as a "breastfeeding couple" for 15 years. Martha has breastfed each of our seven children and is still breastfeeding our 21-month-old at this writing. Many of the self-help techniques we recommend in this book we have learned during our years of experience as co-directors of the Breastfeeding Center in San Clemente, California; Martha has learned additional techniques while working at the Lactation Institute in Encino, California, one of the primary breastfeeding education centers in the world. Much of the material is also based on our personal experience in counseling breastfeeding mothers for the past 20 years. Our goal in writing this book is not only to promote breastfeeding, but even more importantly, to help both baby and mother enjoy this beautiful relationship.

William and Martha Sears
San Clemente, California
1991

1

PRENATAL PREPARATION FOR BREASTFEEDING

Just as prenatal preparation for birth gives you a greater chance of enjoying your baby's birth, the same preparation for breastfeeding increases the likelihood of you and your baby enjoying this relationship.

We advise all first-time breastfeeding mothers to avail themselves of the following prenatal experiences.

Join La Leche League International (LLLI). This is an international volunteer organization composed of women members and group leaders, all of whom strongly advocate breastfeeding. Each leader, besides having practical breastfeeding experience, has special training in counseling new mothers about common concerns of child care. They have access to a lending library, a board of medical consultants, and continuing input from other members through monthly meetings, approximately 13,000 league leaders and 4,200 groups in 45 countries. Although LLLI's motto is "Good Mothering through Breastfeeding," the philosophy of this group is simply good mothering in all aspects of child care.

When you join, you participate in an international mother-to-mother helping network, a valuable resource for parenting help and support. Your annual dues include a magazine filled with stories, breastfeeding tips, and inspiration from other breastfeeding families. Members receive a discount on books and publications on breastfeeding, childbirth, nutrition, and parenting. Your membership also helps to support La Leche League International work. For more information, see the Resources List on page 168

Before your baby is born attend four monthly La Leche League meetings. These get-togethers, held in a member's home, cover all aspects of breastfeeding, right start techniques, the effect of breastfeeding on the family, and practical tips on making breastfeeding a more enjoyable experience. Besides being informative, they help you meet mothers who may be of valuable support after the baby is born.

Choose health care providers who are knowledgeable about breastfeeding. When making the rounds to choose doctors for yourself and your baby, choose a health care professional who is knowledgeable and supportive of breastfeeding, not one who only gives lip service to it. What is the percentage of breastfeeding mothers in your practice? How long do you think mothers should breastfeed? How would you treat sore nipples and handle breastfeeding problems? What would you do if our baby wasn't gaining enough weight on my milk? Is there a lactation consultant in your practice or do you work closely with one? Are mothers encouraged to join La Leche League? You want the prospective doctor to know that breastfeeding is a high priority in your overall parenting style. In our Breastfeeding Center, we have seen many failures due to improper advice or lack of encouragement. Any advice that shakes the confidence of a new mother can undermine the whole breastfeeding relationship.

Take a breastfeeding class. These classes are offered as part of the package by most hospital childbirth classes. These classes will instruct you on preparation for breastfeeding, right start techniques, and how to prevent and overcome the most common breastfeeding difficulties. As part of your prenatal breastfeeding education it is wise to get in touch with a lactation consultant (this may even be your class instructor). This is a relatively new specialty in the field of childcare. There are training programs throughout the country that offer a one- to two-year course on becoming a lactation consultant, and one can now obtain a master's degree in this specialty; the most experienced of these programs is the Lactation Institute, Encino, California. To select a lactation consultant, look for the credentials IBCLC—International Board of Certified Lactation Consultants.

Prepare your breasts. Many lactation specialists believe that most women do not need much breast preparation; sore nipples are avoided primarily by correct positioning and latch-on after baby arrives,rather than by specific preparation before birth.

To prepare for baby's vigorous sucking, consider the following prenatal care for your nipples. Avoid using soap on your breasts, as this may dry the skin and encourage nipple cracking. Rinsing with plain water when you bathe will keep the nipple clean. Glands around your nipple secrete a natural lubricating substance, so lotions and oils are not necessary. Some nursing mothers have toughened their nipples by going without a bra for part of the day or by wearing a nursing bra with the flaps down and exposing the nipples to the air and the light friction of clothing.

Breast massage will help you become more comfortable in handling your breasts, and it is a technique you may find useful when expressing your milk later on (see Key 6).

Have your nipples examined prenatally by a health care provider knowledgeable in recognizing flat or inverted nipples. Breastfeeding gets off to a smoother start if baby has a graspable nipple to latch onto. Some women, however, have flat or inverted nipples, which make latch-on somewhat difficult. Baby's efforts to compensate can lead to sore nipples. Flat or inverted nipples are easy to detect and manage. During the first trimester of your pregnancy, check the response of your nipples to this simple test. Place your thumb and index finger on the edges of the areola (the dark portion of your breast, surrounding the nipple) and press in as much as you can, gently but firmly. The nipple should remain erect or project further outward. If, instead, your nipple flattens or retracts (inverts) into the breast, you should begin wearing breast shields about halfway through your pregnancy to gradually draw out the nipple. It is important to do this test, because you cannot tell if you have flat or inverted nipples just by looking. Some nipples appear normal but actually invert when this test is performed. Breast shields (not nipple shields; these are different) are plastic cups that fit inside your bra, placing slight pressure over the areola and allowing the nipple to protrude through a specially designed opening. These, as well as other breastfeeding aids, can be obtained from your local lactation consultant or from La Leche League.

Besides preparing your body for breastfeeding, it is equally important to prepare your mind. Many women are not prepared for the fact that breastfeeding is a lifestyle, a commitment in time, energy, and perseverance during those early weeks when "all the baby wants to do is nurse." As one mother in our practice put it, "Intellectually I was prepared for breastfeeding; emotionally I was not." This mother understood that breast milk was best for her baby and for that reason wanted to breastfeed; but she did not realize the level of commitment it would take during those first few weeks to get over the hump and then to settle down to a more harmonious breastfeeding style. It helps to surround yourself with mothers who enjoy their breastfeeding experience. They will encourage you through those early weeks.

Choose your childbirthing environment wisely. Mothers who have had a stressful and traumatic labor and delivery have a higher incidence of breastfeeding problems. Mothers who have had a caesarean birth also have a higher incidence of unsuccessful breastfeeding, primarily because babies and mothers are separated more, the early harmony is not achieved, and much of the energy needed for breastfeeding is diverted to the healing of mother's own body. Anything you can do to increase your chances of having an uncomplicated childbirth increases your chances of having an uncomplicated breastfeeding relationship. Unless you have particular obstetrical risks, choose an LDR room (mother labors, delivers, and recovers in the same room). Besides taking a good natural childbirth class, employ the services of a labor support person, a woman trained in either childbirth instruction or midwifery who can be with you throughout your labor and encourage you to move with the flow of your body. Studies have shown that mothers who are tended by labor support persons progress better in their labors; the presence of the labor support person frees the husband to give emotional support to his wife. Laboring in water also helps mothers progress, as the buoyancy of the water enhances relaxation. Spending a lot of time on your back in bed and not moving with the flow of your body during labor slows down labor and is one of the common reasons for "failure to progress" and consequent caesarean section. How a baby and mother get started with each other during labor often sets the tone for how they will get started with breastfeeding.

2

UNDERSTANDING HOW YOUR BREASTS PRODUCE MILK

To better understand the value of proper breastfeeding technique and appreciate the womanly art of breastfeeding, it helps to understand how your breasts produce milk. The lactation system inside your breast resembles a tree. The glandular tissues are the leaves where the milk is produced; the ducts are the branches where the milk moves down into what will be the trunk of the tree, called the **milk sinuses,** which are the reservoirs where the milk collects waiting to be released into baby's mouth through the nipple. These milk sinuses are located beneath the **areola** (the dark area surrounding your nipple). Milk empties from the sinuses to approximately 15 to 20 openings in your nipple. To effectively empty these milk sinuses, your baby's gums must be positioned *over* them so that his jaws compress the sinuses where the milk is pooled. As we will mention many times throughout this book, babies suck areolas, not nipples. If baby sucks only on your nipple, little milk will be drawn out and your nipple will be traumatized unnecessarily. Baby should have at least one inch of your areola all the way around the nipple in his mouth.

When your baby sucks, the nerve endings in your nipples stimulate the pituitary gland in your brain to secrete the hormone prolactin. This hormone stimulates your milk glands to continue milk production. The first milk the baby receives at each feeding is the **foremilk,** which is thin, like skim milk, because of its low fat content. As your baby continues suckling, the nerve endings in the nipple stimulate the pituitary gland to secrete another hormone called oxytocin. This hormone causes the tissue around your milk glands to contract like a rubber band and squeeze a large supply of milk from the milk glands into the sinuses. This latter milk, or **hindmilk,** is much higher in fat and slightly higher in protein, and, therefore, has greater nutritional value. The hindmilk is the primary nutrient for your infant's growth. Most mothers have a tingling sensation in their breasts as the hindmilk is ejected from the milk glands into the milk sinuses. This sudden outpouring of hindmilk is called the **letdown reflex** because of the "letting down" of the creamier milk.

Because I find the older term "letdown reflex" somewhat depressing, we will use the term "milk ejection reflex." A successful **milk ejection reflex** is the fundamental key to successful breastfeeding. This reflex is characterized by a feeling of fullness or tingling that occurs 30 to 60 seconds or more after baby has started suckling and may occur several times during the feeding. Mothers experience this milk ejection reflex in different intensities at different times. Most first time mothers will begin to experience the reflex by the second or third week after beginning breastfeeding. Some mothers never feel it but may recognize it by the leaking that occurs. Your milk-releasing mechanism can be inhibited by fear, tension, pain, or fatigue. These emotions may result in a faulty milk ejection reflex, in which case your infant receives mostly foremilk, which is insufficient in nutrition and satisfaction.

Milk production works on the supply-and-demand principle. The more your infant sucks correctly, the more milk you will produce, until you have both negotiated a proper balance. Your baby develops a "timer" to his feedings, and your breasts and pituitary gland also develop an automatic timer synchronized to your baby's timer. For example, a mother may feel a milk ejection reflex (her timer) at the same time her baby cries for a feeding, although the two may be miles apart. Breastfeeding problems occur when this timer and the supply-and-demand relationship is upset.

How your infant sucks. Aroused by the touch of your nipple to his lips and the scent or taste of your milk, your infant's lips grasp the areola of your breast and his tongue draws your nipple into his mouth and against the rear palate. Your infant's lips and gums compress the areola and underlying milk sinuses, pushing milk toward the nipple. The infant's lips and large suck pads in the cheeks provide an effective seal, creating negative pressure in the mouth. (After a week or two of sucking, you may notice a callouslike growth on your baby's upper lip. These are normal sucking pads, which develop to help your baby latch on more effectively.) The infant's tongue "milks" the areola in a rhythmic motion, delivering milk through the nipple toward the back of the tongue; little squirts of milk are then swallowed. Sucking milk from a bottle through a rubber nipple is a very different suck-swallow process. The difference between sucking actions required on breast and bottle nipples may lead to **nipple confusion** if baby is given bottles during the first few weeks when he is learning to suck properly.

3

ADVANTAGES OF BREASTFEEDING FOR THE BABY

In your baby's first year you will spend more time feeding him than in any other parent-baby interaction. It is important to enjoy this relationship. Breastfeeding has the following advantages for baby and for mother:

1. Human milk is biologically specific for human babies. Every species of mammal formulates a milk that is unique for the nutritional requirements of its offspring. This milk is perfect for each species in order to insure the adaptation of the species to its environment. Each species of animal makes a milk that is high in those particular nutrients that insure the survival of that species. For example, seal milk is high in fat because seals need high body fat to adapt to their cold environment. The milk of cows and other range mammals is high in minerals and protein because rapid bone and muscle growth is necessary for their mobility and survival; the calf is up and running within hours after birth. What is the human survival organ? The brain. Amazingly, human milk is high in specific nutritional elements that promote brain growth. Only recently have scientists been discovering more and more elements in human milk that are unique to the human species.
2. Breast milk is a dynamic living tissue that changes to

meet the nutritional needs of the baby and to protect against disease. It contains living cells, and its nutritional content changes from day to day and hour to hour according to the needs of your baby. An example of this dynamic process is a change in your milk's fat content. Fat accounts for a large percentage of your milk's calories. If your baby is hungry, he feeds in such a way as to get milk with higher fat content. If your baby is only thirsty, he feeds in such a way that he receives a lower-calorie milk. The fat content in your milk changes throughout the day. Your milk gradually becomes lower in fat as your baby gets older because he will need fewer calories per pound of body weight.

Your milk also changes to protect your baby against germs. Your baby needs a supply of germ-fighting elements in his blood, **immunoglobulins.** Shortly after birth the infant begins making his own immunoglobulins, but they do not reach sufficient levels to protect him until he is about six months old. To make up for this deficiency, the mother gives her baby her immunoglobulins through her milk until he is able to make his own. Even after six months, breast milk continues to supply immunoglobulins. If a mother is exposed to a germ, her milk provides her baby with antibodies that protect him from the same germ. The white cells in mother's milk also produce a special protein that coats the baby's intestines, preventing the passage of harmful germs from his intestines into his blood.

The very first milk your baby receives shortly after birth is called **colostrum.** This milk provides heavy doses of disease immunity. Since your newborn baby is particularly vulnerable to germs, your milk is the most protective when your baby needs it most.

3. Human milk contains just the right amount of the six nutrients that baby needs: fat, protein, carbohydrates, minerals, iron, and vitamins.

Fats. Your milk contains enzymes to help the fat be digested completely. Because formula does not contain these enzymes, the fat in formula or cow's milk is not totally digested and some passes into the stools, accounting for the unpleasant odor of the stools of formula-fed infants. Breast milk contains cholesterol; formula does not. I am greatly concerned about taking cholesterol out of formulas because it is fashionable to have low cholesterol diets—for **adults.** Surely it is no mistake that the oldest living recipe for human nutrition contains cholesterol. Could it be that the cholesterol in breast milk helps the infant's liver learn to process cholesterol and thus protects the child against higher cholesterol later on? Nutritionists are still not in agreement about this cholesterol question, but common sense suggests that nature would not make an error.

Protein. The curd produced from your milk is smaller and more digestible than that of cow's milk or formula, which is why mothers have observed that the formula-fed baby remains "full" longer than the breastfed baby. Because breast milk contains only human proteins, it is naturally less allergenic than formulas containing proteins from other species or vegetable proteins.

Carbohydrates. The predominant sugar in breast milk is lactose. Researchers have noted that mammals with larger brains have a larger percentage of lactose in their milk. Human milk contains more lactose than cow's milk; that is why it tastes sweeter. To make the sweetness similar to mother's milk, cane sugar and corn syrup are added to some formulas, but all sugars are not the same. Cane sugar is digested more rapidly than lactose, and we know that some older children have mood swings when they eat cane sugar. Perhaps infants also have blood sugar swings when eating cane sugar in formula.

Lactose favors the development of certain beneficial bacteria in your baby's intestines. These bacteria ward off other bacteria that cause diarrhea. The combination of the artificial, acid-forming sugars and the excess fat in the stools of formula-fed babies often accounts for the "acid burn" diaper rash that is common among them.

Minerals. Cow's milk is high in calcium and phosphorus because cows have a much higher rate of bone growth than humans. These excess mineral salts add an extra load to your infant's immature kidneys. Human milk is lower in mineral salts and therefore easier on your newborn's kidneys.

Iron. Your baby needs iron to make new blood cells as he grows. As the baby was developing in the womb, he received a lot of iron from your blood through the placenta. He uses up these iron stores within his first six months; therefore, he needs extra iron. The iron in your breast milk is different from any other kind of iron. Babies who are fed breast milk very rarely become anemic, whereas babies fed cow's milk or formula without iron often become anemic between one and two years of age. The amount of iron in formula and in breast milk has entirely different effects on a baby. Your baby can absorb only ten percent of the iron in iron-fortified formula and cereals, compared to at least 50 percent of the iron in breast milk. The reason for this difference is a special protein in your milk called **lactoferrin.** This special substance attaches to the iron in your milk and helps your baby's intestine absorb the iron, thus protecting your baby against anemia. The excess iron in formula, however, is excreted in the stools. This accounts for the green color of formula-fed baby's stool. A baby's stool neither looks right nor smells right when his intestines are called upon to handle milk they are not designed to handle. Excess iron in the intestines also allows the growth of harmful bacteria that can cause diarrhea.

Vitamins. Breast milk contains all the essential vitamins that your baby needs, so vitamin supplements are not necessary in breastfed infants. All the vitamins, minerals, iron, carbohydrates, fats, and proteins have been adapted over centuries to insure the optimal survival of the young of the species.

Because breast milk is the perfect nutrient, long ago mother's milk was known as "white blood." Breastfed infants often have more comfortable bowel movement patterns. Colostrum, your baby's first milk, has a natural laxative effect that clears the sticky meconium, or fetal waste matter, from your baby's intestines during the first week. Breastfed stools are more frequent, less odorous, softer, and easier to pass.

4. Breastfeeding benefits babies' oral-facial development. Your newborn's oral-facial construction is uniquely adapted to breastfeeding. His upper lip con-

tains a blisterlike "sucking pad." His rounded cheeks are filled with abundant fat pads, his tongue is oversized and his palate is arched. All these physical characteristics are designed to fit the contour of your breast. The facial and tongue muscles work very differently when breastfeeding and when bottle feeding. A breastfed infant sucks more vigorously and orients the milk toward the back of his tongue and palate. He controls the flow of milk better. A bottle-fed infant sucks with the front of his mouth. Orthodonists believe that breastfeeding contributes to the proper alignment of the infant's jawbone, whereas bottle feeding may contribute to malocclusion.

5. The physical advantages to the baby are impressive enough, but when you look at the emotional advantages to mother and baby, the case for breastfeeding is overwhelming. Studies have shown that skin-to-skin contact and touching benefits baby's physical, mental, and emotional development. Fresh from the tension of birth, a baby put to his mother's breast has no separation from his matrix (his safe place)—he hears the familiar heartbeat, the familiar breathing, the familiar voice. He feels the enveloping warmth and touch of her body; his mouth has a place to suck that helps the tension subside. Mother's face is right there, just the right distance, hovering 8 to 12 inches from baby's face—the distance that newborns can see best—so his eyes can drink in who she is, even as he drinks in the colostrum. He is secure, he is home, all is well.

4

ADVANTAGES OF BREASTFEEDING FOR THE MOTHER

The nutritional, physical, and emotional advantages for the baby have been popularized extensively in order to promote breastfeeding throughout the world. The advantages to the mother, however, are often overlooked, and these are really impressive. Mothers may initially feel that breastfeeding is all giving, giving, giving. One of the themes throughout Barron's Parenting Keys is the mutual giving that occurs between parent and baby. This is best illustrated in the breastfeeding relationship. Mother gives baby her milk and baby "gives" something back to the mother. Every time baby sucks from her breast, he causes a hormone called **prolactin** to be released into her bloodstream. This is the magical substance that travels throughout the highways of mother's body telling her which turn to take.

The prolactin stimulation from breastfeeding is especially helpful for some mothers. They sincerely love their babies but do not feel they will have the "mother's intuition" that everybody tells them they should have. The hormonal stimulation provided by breastfeeding gets these mothers started.

Breastfeeding helps the mother's body adjust to changes after birth. As the newborn sucks from her breast, the hormone oxytocin is released, which causes the uterus to return to its normal shape more quickly. When baby is put to the breast immediately after birth, this natural hormone hastens the delivery of the placenta and the clamping down on uterine blood vessels, minimizing blood loss.

Breastfeeding is important for the busy lifestyles of today's mothers. Mothers in our practice who work outside the home will often relate that when they come home from a hectic day's work, as soon as they nurse their babies they feel relaxed. A prime example of both the relaxing and mutual giving effects of breastfeeding is how breastfeeding helps mothers sleep. Mother gives baby her milk, which contains a recently discovered sleep-inducing substance to help baby sleep. The baby's sucking stimulates the relaxing hormones to come into mother. Mother helps put the baby to sleep and the baby helps put the mother to sleep. This is especially beneficial for busy mothers who have trouble napping and sleeping. Because breastfed babies need to be fed more often, this method of feeding in some ways "forces" the mother to sit down, relax, and nurse. It seems as if nature provides a feeding system that encourages the mother to take proper care of herself. A bottle-feeding mother can seemingly carry on a busier lifestyle because someone else can feed the baby, but this is what wears out mothers.

Many mothers find that the instant availability and proper temperature of the milk (especially at night and while traveling) make breastfeeding less time-consuming and difficult than preparing formula.

Breastfeeding contributes to mother's health. There is a lower incidence of breast cancer in women who have breastfed. This may be an important consideration if there is a strong family history of cancer.

Breastfeeding promotes natural child spacing. While not a foolproof method of contraception, breastfeeding does suppress ovulation in most women. (See Key 34 for Breastfeeding as a Natural Contraceptive.)

Breastfeeding also has economic benefits. Your baby will probably be healthier, so you will have fewer medical and dental bills. In addition, you will save money by not buying formulas and as much canned baby foods.

Breastfeeding mothers have one free hand with which to mother another sibling or two. A mother who is breastfeeding a newborn can read a story to a toddler—or just sit and cuddle. This can go a long way toward easing the toddler's feelings of being left out, while presenting a beautiful, natural life process to other family members.

One of the main benefits of breastfeeding to the mother that we have noticed in our practice is how much in harmony a breastfeeding mother is with her infant. She seems to go more with the flow of the infant, reading her baby's cues and responding appropriately; the two seem to be in sync. This later translates into having a comfortable knowledge of the child. There is great comfort in really knowing and understanding your child. Breastfeeding gives this bonding a head start.

We have only skimmed the surface in mentioning the primary advantages of breastfeeding for baby, mother, and family. It seems that every month in the medical journals we read another exciting discovery about the unique properties of human milk for human babies. Science is only now beginning to discover what mothers have known all along—that something good happens to babies and mothers when they breastfeed.

5

RIGHT START TECHNIQUES

Studying mothers at our Breastfeeding Center who have successfully breastfed their babies, we have put together the following recipe for getting the right start.

1. **Breastfeed immediately after birth.** Unless a medical condition prevents it, your first breastfeeding can occur just minutes after baby's birth, and both baby and mother will benefit. This is the time when baby will be in a state of quiet alertness and very receptive toward sucking. After his initial cries are soothed, he will gaze around, searching for your face and eyes and reaching out with his mouth for your breast. Guide his movement and let him nuzzle your nipple, looking and making his first attempts to suck. This first nursing is important for several reasons. The first milk you produce, called colostrum, is the best food for him now; the sooner baby starts, the better. Sucking helps the newly delivered baby to ease the tension built up from the stress of labor and birth. Sucking is a familiar and comforting function—babies suck in the womb—so it helps baby adjust to his new environment. Most importantly, this first sucking at the breast is baby's first lesson in breastfeeding, given at a time of optimal receptivity. In just an hour or two your baby will want to sleep, and this sleepiness may last off and on for several days.

2. **Position yourself properly.** If you are able, sitting up in a bed or rocking chair is the easiest position for nursing. Pillows are a real must. Place one behind your back, one on your lap for your baby, and another under the arm that will support your baby. Get comfortable before beginning to nurse. Relaxation is needed for the milk ejection reflex to occur. If sitting in a chair, use a footstool under your feet to elevate your lap and get baby closer to your breast.

3. **Position baby properly.** Undress your baby to promote skin-to-skin contact. This keeps him from falling asleep and helps him suck better. Nestle baby in your arms so that his neck rests in the bend of your elbow, his back along your forearm and his buttocks in your hand. Turn baby's entire body so that he is facing you tummy to tummy. His head should be straight, not arched backward or turned sideways in relation to the rest of his body. The baby should not have to turn his head or strain his neck to reach your nipple. Turn your head to the side or up to the ceiling and try to swallow! Baby must also be up at the level of your breast, so you will need a pillow or two on your lap. (If sitting, it helps to raise your lap more by putting your feet on a footstool.) If you try to hold baby up with your arms, your back and arm muscles will be strained. If baby rests low on your lap, he will be pulling down on your breasts, causing unnecessary stretching and friction. Bring baby up and in toward you rather than leaning forward toward baby; it is much easier on your back. As you turn baby on his side, tuck his lower arm into the soft pocket between baby and your midriff, bending him so that he is wrapped around you tummy to tummy. If his upper arm keeps interfering with latch-on, you can hold it

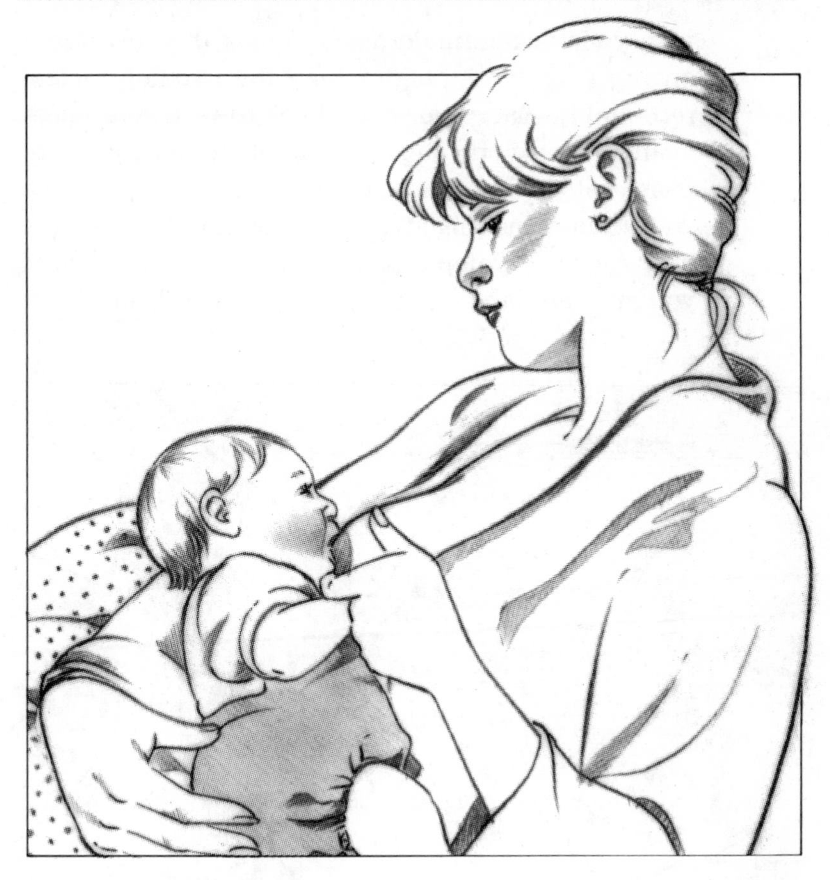

down with the thumb of your hand that is holding baby. This basic position is called the cradle hold. If you have a small baby or experience difficulty with the following latch-on sequence, go immediately to using the clutch hold or position described in point 6.

4. **Present your breast.** With your free hand, manually express a few drops of milk to moisten your nipple. Cup your breast, supporting the weight of your breast

with your fingers underneath, and with your thumb on top (this works better than the two-finger cigarette hold). Place your hand back toward your chest wall to keep your fingers clear of the areola, away from baby's latch-on site. Be sure not to pinch your thumb and fingers together tightly, because this may cause the nipple to retract in some breasts. If you are very large-breasted, use a rolled hand towel

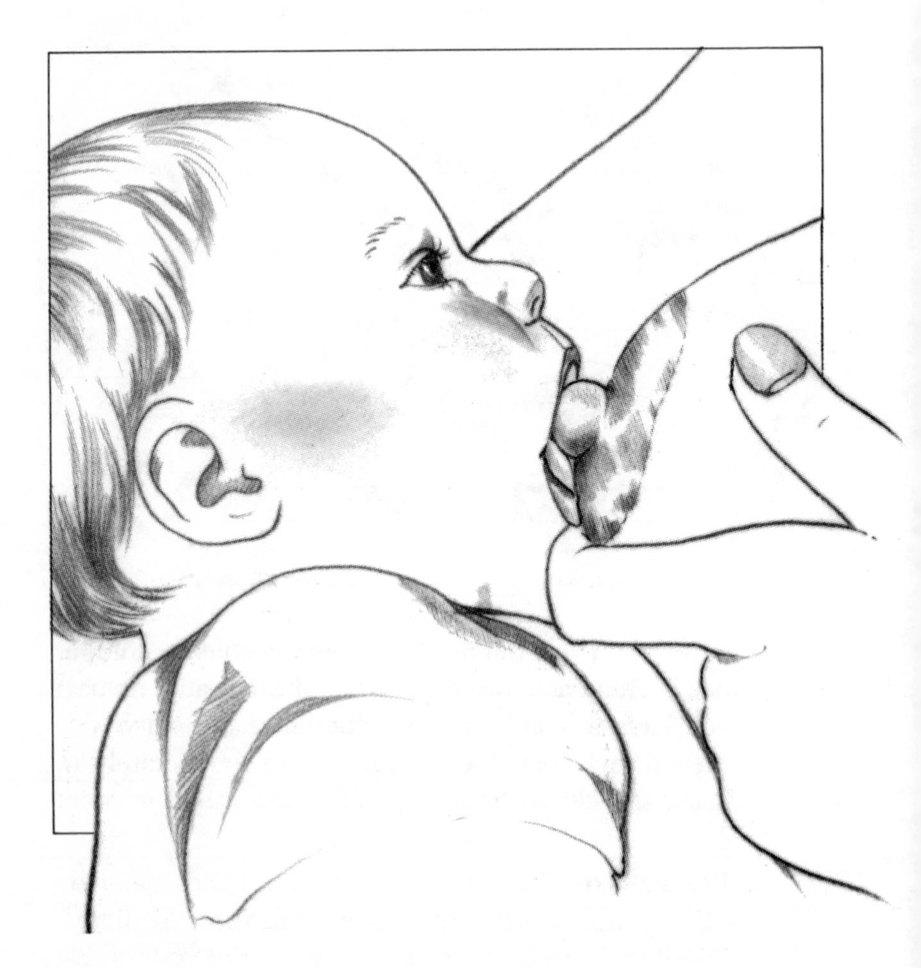

under your breast to support its weight so that it doesn't drag down on baby's lower jaw and tire his mouth.

5. **Encourage proper latch-on—the most important step.** Gently tickle baby's lips with your milk-moistened nipple as a teaser. Encourage baby to open his mouth widely (babies' mouths open like little birds' beaks—very wide—and then quickly close). The moment your baby opens his mouth widely, direct your nipple into his mouth (be sure to place it above his tongue), and with a **rapid** movement pull him **very close** to you with the arm that is holding him. This technique is known as R.A.M. (Rapid Arm Movement). Don't lean forward, pushing your breast toward your baby; pull him toward you. Most new mothers do not pull their babies close enough. Attempt to get a large part of your areola into his mouth. Maximize the amount of areola in his mouth **by flanging his lips outward;** do not allow him to tighten his lips inward. This is done by pulling down on his chin and, using your finger, flanging his lower lip outward. (In teaching breastfeeding techniques to nurses and interns, we frequently make "lower lip rounds." By simply pulling the lower jaw down a bit and flanging the tight, inwardly turned lower lip, mothers exclaim, "It doesn't hurt anymore; it feels right.") The key to correct latch-on is for your baby to grasp onto the areola, the dark area of your breasts surrounding your nipple. Under the areola are the milk sinuses, which should be compressed for proper milk release. Pull your baby so close that the tip of his nose touches your breast. Don't be afraid of blocking his nose, since he can breathe quite well from the sides of his nose even if the tip is compressed. If baby's nose does seem to be

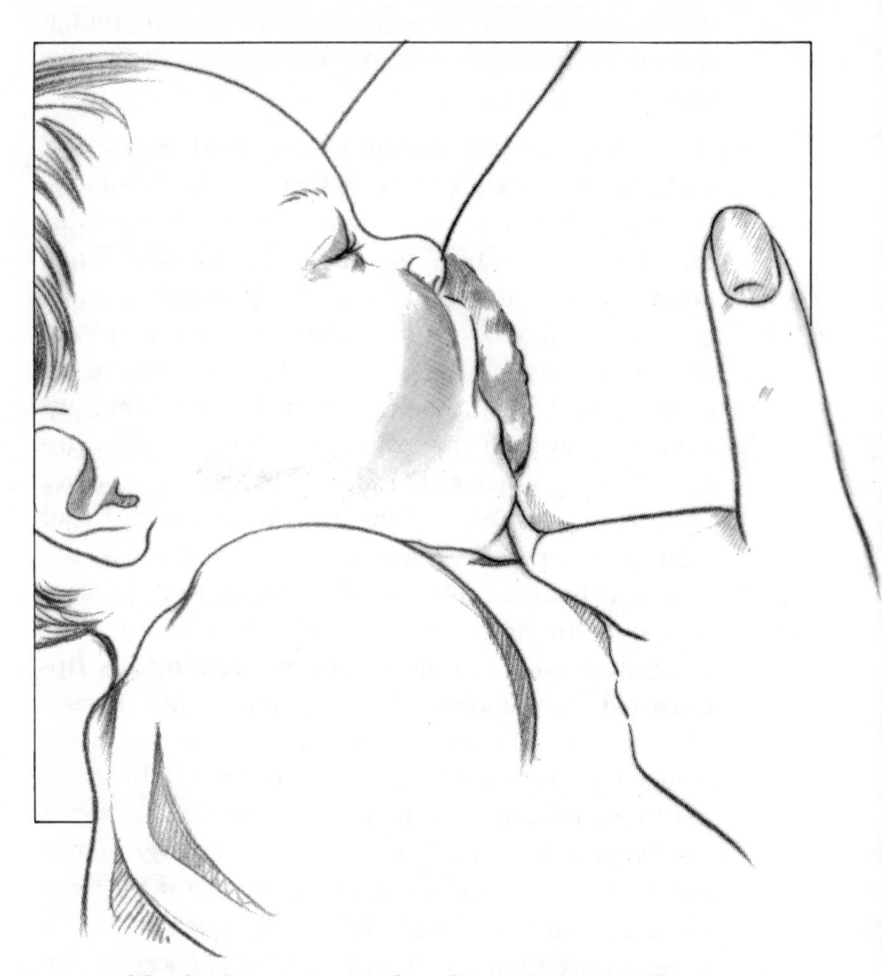

blocked, use your thumb to press gently on your breasts to uncover his nose, or simply change the angle of his body slightly by pulling his legs in close. Hold your breast throughout the feeding until baby is old enough to handle the weight of your breast.

If you have flat or inverted nipples or if baby has a weak suck, there is an additional step you need to use. As soon as you have latch-on, as baby starts to suck, compress your breast with your thumb and fingers—this stabilizes the milk ducts and holds them forward so baby does not lose his grasp so easily.

As you R.A.M. baby on, be sure that your nipple is centered in his mouth and that baby does not slide down onto the nipple. His gums should completely bypass the nipple and come to rest about an inch behind the nipple on the areola. If you do it quickly enough, his mouth will close down far back on your areola, not on the nubbin of your nipple. If your baby is latching on correctly, you should not feel painful pressure on your nipple. **Remember, baby should suck the areola, not the nipple.** If baby seems to be latching on incorrectly, you may have to make him stop sucking (break the suction with your finger between his gums) and start over several times until you get it right. Don't allow your baby to continue sucking incorrectly because it hurts and because it is wrong patterning and a habit that is hard to break.

Some babies learn to slide onto the nipple, slurping it in as they go but stopping short of the ideal position. This results in a frustrated baby who gets little milk and a mother who gets sore nipples. If baby persistently clamps down too hard, tell him to "open" while depressing his lower jaw with your finger on his chin. You should notice instant relief from the pain. If your baby does not cooperate, break the suction and start again.

Again, if baby's lips are pursed tightly inward, flange them out. It is important that he learns to latch on the right way. Many babies latch on as a natural instinct, but some babies have to be taught. Babies exhibit various styles; some latch right on and suck like a pro the minute they find the nipple, while others seem more interested in looking around or lazily playing with the nipple. A slow starter who likes to suck a little and snooze a little needs some prodding and needs to be held skin-to-skin in his mother's arms. With constant encouragement, the sleepy baby gradually will suck longer and more enthusiastically.

After a few weeks, you will notice that your baby exhibits two types of sucking: comfort sucking, a weaker suck primarily with the lips in which the baby gets the foremilk; and nutritional sucking, a more vigorous sucking with the tongue and jaw. Notice the muscles of his face working so hard that even his ears wiggle during intense nutritional sucking. This kind of productive sucking rewards your baby with the higher-calorie hindmilk. The visible contractions of the baby's jaw muscles and the audible swallow sounds are reliable indications that your baby has good sucking techniques.

6. **Alternative nursing positions.** Two other basic breastfeeding positions you need to know are the clutch hold and the lying-down position. By varying the way you hold baby to feed him, you will be less likely to get sore nipples because baby's mouth will be putting pressure on different points on the areola. For both these positions, the method of getting baby to latch on is the same as the cradle hold. The lying-down position is basically the cradle hold, but with the baby and mother lying on their sides facing each other. Place two pillows under your head, one behind your back, and another under your top leg, and tuck a fifth pillow behind the baby so your arm doesn't have to continue to hold your baby in close once you

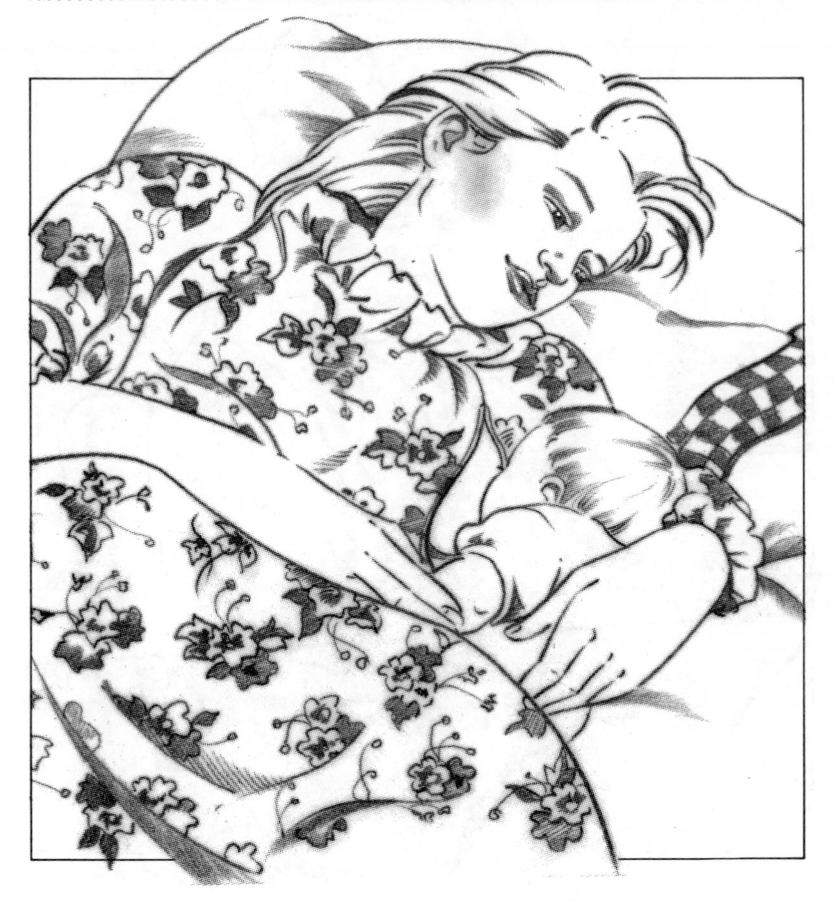

drift off to sleep. Place the baby on his side facing you and nestled in your arm, and slide the baby up or down so his mouth lines up with your nipple. Use the same positioning and latch-on techniques as described above.

7. Another nursing arrangement is the **clutch hold** (football hold). Sitting up in bed or in a comfortable armchair, position baby under your arm along the same

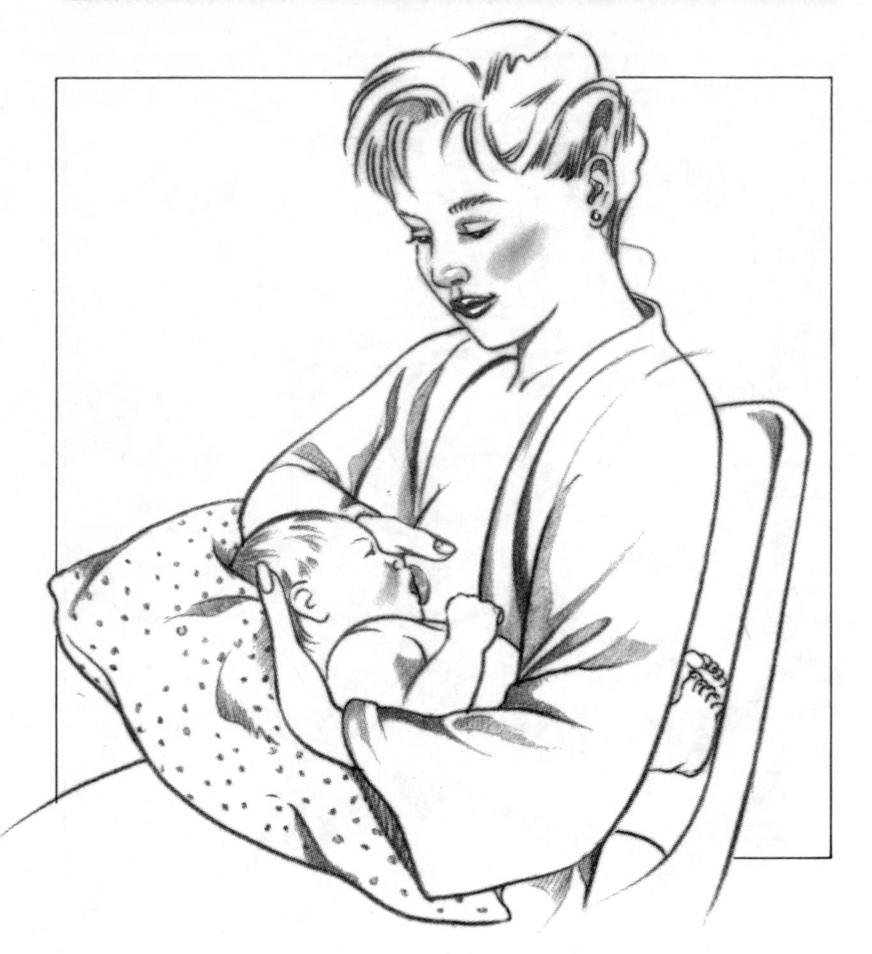

side as the breast you are using. Place a pillow at your side and put the baby on the pillow. Cup the back of his neck in your hand and direct his legs upward so they are resting against the pillow supporting your back. Pull baby in close to you (R.A.M.) and, once baby is sucking well, push a pillow or two against his back to hold him close. Lean back in your bed or chair and enjoy the feeding period. Be sure baby is not pushing with his feet against the back of the chair or pillow, causing him to arch his back. If this happens, position baby bent at his hips with his legs and buttocks up against the chair back. The clutch hold is especially effective for babies who squirm, arch their backs, and frequently detach themselves from the breasts, as well as for small or premature babies, who need more guidance and support from mother's hands.

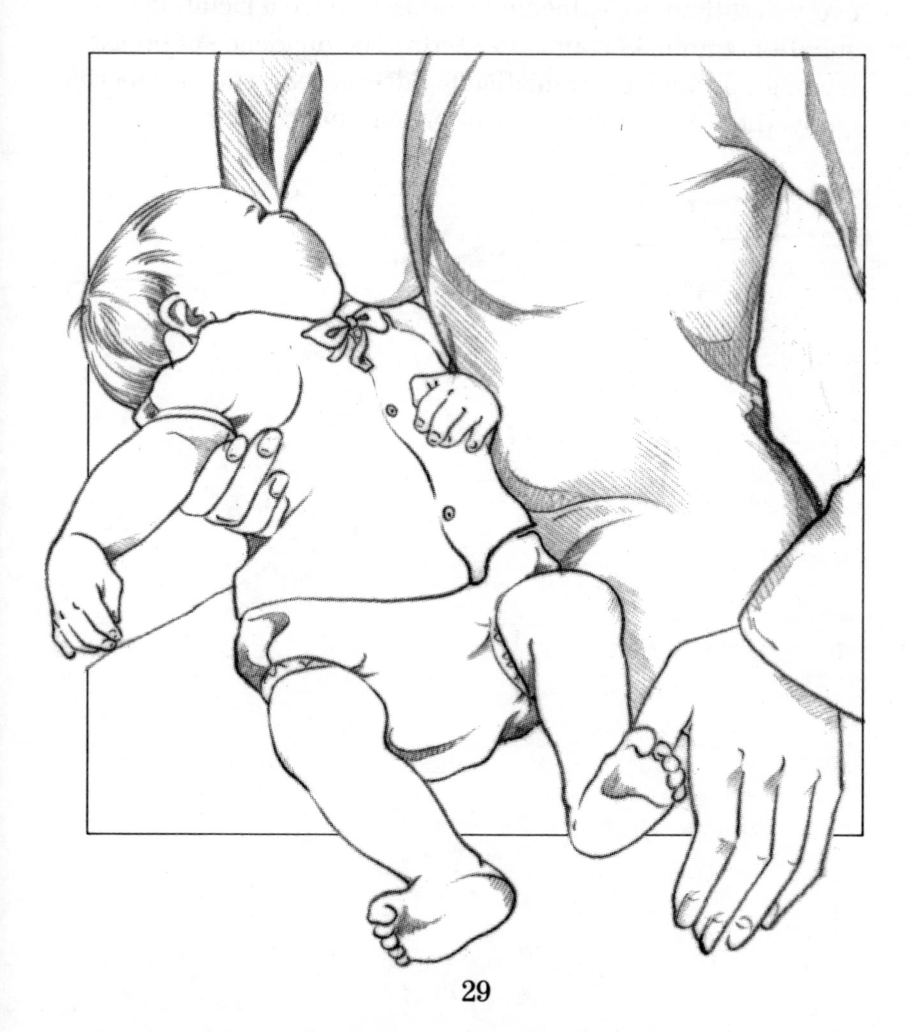

We cannot overemphasize the importance of following the steps of proper positioning and latch-on. Most of the breastfeeding problems we see (sore nipples, insufficient milk, mothers not enjoying breastfeeding) are due to improper positioning and latch-on. It is wise for a first-time breastfeeding mother to seek the services of a lactation specialist within the first several days in order to get a right start with proper position and latch-on before abnormal sucking habits develop. A few years ago in our practice, we started requiring every first-time breastfeeding mother to have a lactation consultation within 48 hours after birth. The incidence of breastfeeding problems dramatically decreased and mothers enjoyed the breastfeeding relationship much more.

6

MANUAL EXPRESSION OF MILK

The techniques for manual expression of breastmilk can be very individual. Martha learned how to do it in 1975 when our third baby was born. Here is how she describes it: When Peter was one month old I was back at work several afternoons a week and I wanted to leave breastmilk for him. I found that I could express between six and eight ounces of milk in about 20 minutes at a break during the afternoon. I learned to do this first at home in order to make my trial and error practice more relaxed. A week or two before, I started to build up a supply by expressing just an ounce or two in the morning when my breasts were the fullest. On the first day back at work I had several four-ounce bottles in the freezer—a little stockpile that gave me some leeway in learning how the routine would work away from home.

Here's how I did it. I locked the door first, washed my hands, and got comfortable. A big drink of water helped me "prime the pump," so to speak, and I thought of my little Peter and the way he was feeding at my breast just a few hours earlier, just before I left him. Before I actually began to express milk I massaged both my breasts at once, which helped to relax me even more and even sometimes activated the milk ejection reflex (MER) so that the milk began dripping. I had a clean plastic bottle as my only tool and I simply directed my nipple into the opening. This was rather awkward, but it worked fine after I got used to it. Medela makes a hand expression funnel that makes it easier to catch the sprays of milk more conveniently (see the list of resources in the back of the book).

I started with the fullest, "drippiest" breast and learned how to press with my forearm against the other nipple to stop the leaking (no sense wasting any of this liquid gold!). Holding the collecting bottle with one hand, I cupped my breast with the other hand. I started with the hand on the same side as the breast, and then switched hands to get different angles in order to empty all the sinuses around the "clock" (that is, with thumb and fingers at 12 and 6 o'clock, then at 10 and 4; then at 2 and 8 with the other hand).

The actual movements of the milking hand become quite rhythmic as the milk begins to flow. Begin with the thumb on top just at the edge of your areola and your other fingers on the other side of the areola directly opposite. You may vary the distance from the nipple that works best for you after you experiment with several positions. The milk sinuses can be felt (and even seen bulging) as they fill up with the MER. Move your thumb and fingers together toward the nipple with just enough firmness to produce a spray of milk; continue to repeat this movement rhythmically. As the MER activates, the milk will often even spray out on its own. When it subsides, go back to the firm, rhythmic movements and continue until milk just dribbles. Change to another position and release more milk, then change hands and go to another position on the areola "clock." By now you've been expressing milk for about 6 to 8 minutes. You can now switch to the second breast and repeat the whole process.

The pamphlet published by La Leche League entitled "Manual Expression of Breastmilk, Marmet Technique" (see list of resources) has a very precise detailed description with illustrations. If you find you're having trouble perfecting your own technique, obtain a copy before you assume you just can't get the knack. This pamphlet has helped thousands of mothers. Even experienced mothers have been able to express more milk. Mothers who were able to express little or none at all have had excellent results.

There are distinct advantages to using a manual technique rather than a mechanical pump:

- Some mothers find some pumps uncomfortable or ineffective.
- Mothers often feel put off by the mechanical gadgetry and prefer the natural approach.
- Skin to skin stimulation can actually produce the milk ejection reflex better.
- Your hands are "handy"—convenient, portable, available, and best of all, free!

7

BREASTFEEDING THE CAESAREAN BABY

Remember that caesarean delivery is primarily a birth, secondarily an operation. It used to be the custom to separate caesarean-birthed babies and mothers for 24 hours while mother recovered from the operation. During this time, baby was given a bottle of water or artificial formula until mother and baby were reunited to begin feeding. Since most mothers are now awake during the caesarean birth (if they have an epidural anesthesia), unless a medical reason prevents it, baby can be placed on mother's chest and nestled right beneath her neck immediately after birth. It usually requires the father to sit there and support baby's weight while the three have a private bonding time. There have even been occasions where I have seen a baby breastfeed right after a caesarean delivery, but this is a bit awkward because of the surgical drapes and may interfere with the sterility of the operation. If you have a caesarean birth and wish to breastfeed, consider the following right start techniques.

1. **Father bonding.** Immediately after birth, while the incision is being closed and mother taken to the recovery room, father can bond with the baby, talking and stroking and singing to his baby in the nursery. As soon as mother is awake, even in the recovery room, the healthy baby can be brought to mother to begin breastfeeding (if baby is stable and mother is able). I have noticed that one of the best pain relievers while recovering from an operation is a frequent "injection" of baby into mother's arms.

The lying-down position and the clutch hold (see Key 5) are usually best for the postoperative caesarean mother, as these positions keep baby's weight off the incision. Because movement will be painful during the first couple of days, you will need a nurse or lactation consultant to help position baby for proper latch-on. The nurse or breastfeeding consultant should also instruct the father on how to help baby latch on, especially holding baby's lower jaw down and flanging baby's lips outward since mother may not be mobile enough to bend over to see how baby is latching on. Don't worry about the effect of pain medication going through your milk. In fact, it is important to use your medication to keep the pain from interfering with your ability to hold and breastfeed your baby. If the postoperative pain medication keeps you from being able to breastfeed for several hours or even a day after birth (this is not usual), father or a nurse can give baby glucose and water or an artificial formula by syringe. The **syringe and finger feeding technique** is superior to use of a bottle, which may lead to nipple confusion.

2. Because of postoperative sedation, rooming-in is usually discouraged for a caesarean mother. It is possible, however, if you are in an LDR room and father or a labor support person rooms-in with you and can comfort and feed baby while you are sleeping.

Keep positive. Many of the energies that would otherwise be directed toward establishing breastfeeding will need to be directed toward the necessary healing of your own body. It usually takes more time to achieve a harmonious breastfeeding relationship following a caesarean than following a less complicated birth, but it is well worth the perseverance.

8

THE IMPORTANCE OF ROOMING-IN

Healthy mothers and healthy babies should be together from birth until discharge from the hospital. Mother is the primary caregiver and the medical personnel assume the roles of helpers and advisors.

Rooming-in allows the breastfeeding pair to get in harmony with each other. When baby gives a cue that he needs food or comfort, mother is immediately there to see and respond to this cue. Baby learns to cue better and trusts that his cues will be responded to; mother learns to respond better and gradually trusts that she is responding appropriately as the nursing pair get in sync with each other.

The cry of a newly born baby is an **attachment-oriented behavior.** It is designed to do something to the listener, especially the mother. In response to your own baby's cry, the blood flow and milk-producing hormones increase in your breasts; this is accompanied by the biological urge to pick up and nurse your baby. Within a day or so, mother learns to read the baby's pre-cry signal so that the baby soon learns he does not have to cry to be picked up and nursed.

Contrast a rooming-in baby with a nursery-cared-for baby. Baby wakes up crying and hungry and is taken to the mother. The mother, meanwhile, has missed the opening scene in this biological drama because she was not present when her baby first cried. By the time baby reaches his mother, she is greeted with more intense, disturbing cries. These disturbing cries often do not trigger the same nurturing and hormonal response in mother. A baby who cries intensely and angrily may not stimulate the breast to prepare for feeding in the way a rooming-in baby does.

Rooming-in allows you to forget the clock.

In our experience we have noticed the following differences between mothers and babies in the rooming-in and non-rooming-in situation:

1. Mother's milk appears 24 to 48 hours sooner in the rooming-in situation.
2. The incidence of breastfeeding problems (sore nipples, engorgement, insufficient milk supply) is much lower in rooming-in mothers.
3. Rooming-in mothers and babies seem to be more in harmony with each other. Rooming-in mothers are well on their way to achieving two important goals of parenting: to know baby and to help baby feel right.
4. Rooming-in mothers experience less postpartum depression.
5. When mother and baby leave the hospital never having been apart since birth, the newborn baby truly knows to whom he or she belongs.

9

"SCHEDULING" THE BREASTFEEDING BABY

Early in your breastfeeding relationship, you will realize that the term "schedule" has absolutely no meaning in breastfeeding a baby. The only schedule a baby will have, and should have, is her own. Listen to your baby's cues and watch your baby, not the clock. We prefer the term "harmony" rather than schedule when referring to the breastfeeding relationship.

Remember, it is the frequency of nursing more than the duration that stimulates your milk-producing hormones. In the first few days most babies suckle in varying intensities, intermittently, and for long periods of time, even as long as an hour. The baby will often fall asleep during a breastfeeding and then wake up in an hour and want to feed again. The duration of feeding often depends upon baby's sucking style. Little gourmets suck gently and intermittently while playing with the nipple and looking around, whereas "barracudas" get down to business quickly and feed ravenously. If your baby is latching on correctly, your nipples will not be traumatized from nursing frequently and long.

Learn to read your baby for signs of hunger and contentment. Breastfeeding cannot be scheduled easily because babies digest breast milk more rapidly than formula; therefore, breastfed babies feel hungry more often and need to be fed more often. Babies also have growth spurts, during which they need more food for more growth. During these growth spurts, expect baby to "marathon" nurse around the clock for a day or so. This is normal and necessary in order to build up milk supply to a higher level and to give baby extra nutrition during the growth spurt. Babies also enjoy periods of extra-nutritive sucking in which they are more interested in the feel than in the food. Sometimes babies are only thirsty and suck a little to obtain some of the watery foremilk. Realistically, expect your baby to breastfeed every two to three hours around the clock for the first month or two.

A dictionary defines harmony as "agreement of feeling, ideas, or actions; getting along well together." This is exactly what the breastfeeding "schedule" is. Schedules are rigid; harmony is flexible. Harmony means you go with the flow of your baby and arrive at a "schedule" that is mutually agreeable to both of you. You will get a real feeling of rightness when you are in sync with your baby. Then you will know that you are on the right schedule.

There is biological and scientific proof that it is good for mothers to breastfeed frequently. Prolactin has a short **half-life.** Every substance that enters the bloodstream dissipates from the blood at a particular rate. The time in which it takes one-half of the substance to disappear from the blood is called its half-life. This biological principle is taken into consideration when doctors prescribe medicine. If a pill has a long half-life, it can be taken once or twice a day; if it has a short half-life it must be taken every four to six hours in order to keep the amount of medicine in the blood at a constant therapeutic level. Prolactin has a half-life of less than an hour. Therefore, if mothers wish to have a constant, high level of it, frequent "doses" of nursing are wise. So when you hear a well-meaning critic say, "All she does is nurse," consider that mother and baby are doing what is biologically correct.

Anthropologists who study infant feeding practices conclude that human infants are designed to be fed frequently day and night. There is a logical reason for this. There are two types of infant care and feeding practices among species:

1. *Intermittent contact species*, such as rabbits, are those that leave the young in secluded nests or burrows while the mother is absent for an extended period of time hunting for food.
2. In *extensive contact species*, the young are carried by, hibernate with or follow the mother day and night at least for the early months.

The differences between these two species types are reflected in the breast milk composition and the interval between feedings. In species with intermittent contact, infants are adapted for separations by receiving their total nutritional requirements in spaced feedings during mother's infrequent visits. The breast milk in these species is high in protein and fat, and feedings take place at widely spaced intervals. In the extensive contact species of mammals (of which humans are one), feedings are frequent (every one to two hours) and milk is *low* in protein and fat. This suggests that the human infant is adapted to frequent feeding and extensive maternal contact. Anthropologists also notice that in cultures that practice the extensive maternal contact style of frequent, around-the-clock feedings, child spacing naturally occurs at three- to five-year intervals. Their conclusion is that the extensive maternal contact pattern has been the norm throughout the history of mankind and that the recent deviation from this time-tested pattern of infant care (scheduled feedings, all night sleeping, and intermittent contact with the infant) may not in fact be the norm.

10

BREASTFEEDING THE PREMATURE OR HOSPITALIZED INFANT

Having a premature infant, particularly if he is sick and in a newborn intensive care unit, can be very stressful to new parents. This is especially true if you have prepared yourself for a beautiful bonding relationship, and instead find yourself separated from your baby for days, weeks, and sometimes even months. The recent advances in newborn intensive care have alleviated this burden somewhat by increasing the chances of taking a healthy baby home from the hospital. But the same technology that is saving more babies has also in some ways displaced mothering, and you may feel totally useless as your baby's caregiver. This feeling can eventually lead to negative feelings about your baby and a spirit of detachment rather than attachment. Parents should be a valuable part of the team caring for the premature baby. Touching your baby a lot and especially breastfeeding can alleviate the common feelings of detachment and insufficient bonding with the premature baby.

Recent research has shown that it is even more important to breastfeed the premature infant. Breast milk provides important infection fighting substances that premature babies lack; such babies need more proteins and calories for "catch up." It has recently been discovered that the milk of mothers who deliver preterm babies is higher in proteins and calories—another example of how the milk of a species adapts for the survival of the young of that species.

Until recent years it was erroneously assumed that a premature baby was too small and weak to breastfeed. It was the custom in most newborn intensive care units not to let a premature baby breastfeed until *after* he was able to tolerate bottle feedings. New research has shown that the opposite is true; premature babies actually do better with breastfeeding than with bottle feeding. These studies indicate that the ability to breastfeed may precede the ability to bottle feed for preterm infants, because the suck-swallow coordination is very different in breast- and bottle feeding. A breastfeeding premature infant tends to suck in bursts of three to five sucks followed by a swallow and a rest. A bottle-feeding premature does not have the rhythmic feeding and pausing that a breastfeeding one does. The energy used by the burst-and-pause method of a breastfeeding infant is less than that used by a bottle feeding. For this reason it has been found that breastfed babies actually grow better, have fewer stop-breathing episodes and tire out less during breastfeeding than with bottle feeding. So not only is breast milk uniquely superior for premature babies, but the way in which the premature baby breastfeeds is beneficial.

Another recent innovation in premature infant care is called *kangaroo care*, an affectionate nickname derived from the easy self-feeding of the baby kangaroo. During kangaroo care, the mother holds her diaper-clad infant underneath her clothing, placing baby in a tummy-to-tummy position between or on her breasts. This allows self-regulatory breastfeeding. Kangaroo care is shown to be particularly beneficial for markedly premature infants, even those as young as 28 weeks. Kangaroo care stimulates the release of the hormones that trigger the milk ejection reflex. Mothers who give kangaroo care are more inclined to breastfeed, produce more milk and breastfeed longer. Studies have shown that they develop a deep attachment to their infants, feel confident about their mothering skills and feel a valuable part of the neonatal intensive care team. Not only does kangaroo care facilitate breastfeeding, but the skin-to-skin contact it provides helps premature babies grow better and leave the hospital sooner.

The therapeutic value of touch and breastfeeding has just recently been recognized. One of the main benefits seems to be that premature infants who spend a great deal of their time skin-to-skin at their mother's breasts have fewer stop-breathing episodes, one of the most common problems in premature babies.

Expect your premature breastfeeding baby to be a very slow feeder. Such babies often suck weakly, tire quickly and fall asleep after only a few minutes of sucking. This is why the term "schedule" is particularly meaningless for premature babies. Prematures should be fed more frequently, almost continuously, for several reasons. Tiny babies have tiny tummies that fill more quickly. Premature babies tire more easily. And premature babies need more calories for catch-up growth. Because premature babies have bizarre sleep and wake schedules, every mother-baby pair must work out a breastfeeding pattern that gets the most milk into the baby without tiring him out.

To understand the important role of the breastfeeding mother in caring for a premature infant, let's go through a typical case of a premature baby who has no respiratory problems but who needs to be in the intensive care unit for "fattening." Here are the steps the breastfeeding mother should consider:

- Rent an electric breast pump and begin pumping your milk as soon as possible after birth. Save this milk and begin feeding it to your baby as soon as he is medically able to take it and by whatever method works best.

- Rather than resorting to the bottle, if the baby is too weak to suck from your breast (and recent experiments show that this is not the problem it is often made out to be), use a supplemental nursing system or the syringe and finger feeding methods described in Key 20.
- Practice kangaroo care. Spend as much time as you can in a rocking chair beside your baby's incubator, with baby wrapped skin-to-skin at your breast. Depending on the policies of the neonatal unit, walk around as much as possible during the kangaroo care, unless your baby is attached to monitoring instruments. The stimulation of your walking motion helps baby breathe more regularly because presumably this is a pattern he was used to in the womb.

Crying keeps premature babies from growing because it wastes oxygen and energy. Breastfeeding, kangaroo care and holding and rocking your baby subdues his crying and hastens his growth. One mother of a very premature baby put it positively: "It is like he is in an outside womb. I have the opportunity of actually seeing his last three months of growth."

- Avoid bottles unless they are medically necessary, as premature babies are particularly prone to nipple confusion. It's better to go from a supplementer system directly on to full breastfeeding, bypassing the bottle stage.

Breastfeeding is particularly valuable for the hospitalized baby. Babies get better quicker and parents feel involved as valuable members of the medical team. Breastfeeding is particularly helpful for infants who are hospitalized for breathing problems, such as croup or bronchitis. In these conditions an upset baby leads to more upset in breathing. On many occasions during my pediatric practice I have seen a mother lean over the crib and breastfeed a baby who is having breathing difficulty, and this relaxes the baby. As baby relaxes, his breathing problem relaxes. The breastfeeding mother saves the baby a lot of uncomfortable medical treatments.

Breastfeeding is also particularly valuable for the infant with a diarrheal illness. Inflamed intestines (called gastroenteritis) cannot tolerate artificial formula but they generally can tolerate breast milk. We have seen many infants with gastroenteritis continue to breastfeed and not become dehydrated, whereas their formula-feeding counterparts with the same illness may wind up in the hospital with dehydration and need intravenous feedings. Chalk up another bonus for mother's milk.

During illness an infant will often revert back into a more primitive and familiar pattern of self-comforting, such as thumbsucking and curling up in a fetal position. Being breastfed while sick lessens the anxiety of hospitalization by helping the infant latch onto a comfortable and pleasurable pattern that he has learned to love and trust.

11

HOW TO TELL IF YOUR BABY IS GETTING ENOUGH MILK

Sometime in your breastfeeding career you will worry whether your baby is getting enough milk. This is part of loving your baby.

In the first week, how your baby's stools change gives you a clue to how much milk he is getting. Normally a baby's stool should go from sticky black to green to brown; then, as soon as your rich, creamy hindmilk appears, stools will become more yellow. A stool that is like yellow mustard, seedy, and having the not unpleasant aroma of buttermilk is one sign that your newborn is getting sufficient quantities of hindmilk. Besides the characteristics of the stools, the number is important. In the first month or two a baby who is getting enough will usually have at least two or three yellow, seedy stools a day. Some breastfed babies may even have a stool during or following each feeding. Some babies will normally only have a stool every two or three days and **if all the other parameters of growth are normal** then this does not signify insufficient milk. Because breast milk has a natural laxative effect, the stools of breastfed babies are more frequent than those of formula-fed babies, which tend to be firmer and darker, with an unpleasant odor. While the stools of a breastfed baby are usually mustard yellow, an occasional green stool is of no consequence if baby seems generally well.

Baby's weight gain is another index of sufficient nutrition. Breastfed babies usually show a slower weight gain than formula-fed babies during the first two weeks; thereafter, breastfed and bottle-fed babies show similar weight gains, averaging about an ounce a day during the last two weeks of the first month. Most babies will gain an average of a pound to a pound and a half during the first month, and an average of a pound and a half each month thereafter for the first six months. They usually grow about an inch a month in length during the first six months. This growth rate is an average, somewhat depending on baby's body type. Long, slender babies (ectomorph body type) may gain less in weight and more in height, whereas endomorphs (short and wide) may gain more in weight than height, and mesomorphs (medium build) may show the "average" weight and height gain mentioned above.

Your baby's skin and appearance will give you an idea of whether or not he is getting enough milk. It is not only the volume of breast milk that is important for good nutrition; it is also the quality. Some babies get enough volume of breast milk, as evidenced by wetting the average amount of diapers each day (six to eight wet cloth diapers, four to five paper diapers), but they may not be getting enough calories. Although they are happy, active, and not dehydrated, such babies are recognized by the looseness of their skin, somewhat scrawny muscle development and diminished fat tissue. These babies get enough volume of milk but do not get the high-quality hindmilk. This is a hindmilk problem, usually manifested by insufficient weight gain but without signs of dehydration. A baby with these characteristics is called a "failure-to-thrive baby"—one who is not getting enough nutrition to thrive. Ways to increase the volume and calorie content of your milk are described in Key 13.

There is also a condition called the "normal slow–weight gaining baby." Some babies, because of their individual metabolism and body type, show a slow but steady weight gain and stay near the bottom of the weight chart but with normal length. If all other conditions are met and baby is doing well, for some this is a normal growth curve.

How your breasts feel before and after feedings will give you another clue to milk supply. Your breasts should feel full before and less full after feedings, and should sometimes leak between feedings. Most mothers will also experience a milk ejection reflex during feedings. (Some normal breastfeeding mothers do not always feel a milk ejection reflex, nor do they always leak.) You may also notice the changing characteristics of your milk. The lower-calorie foremilk is thinner, resembling skim milk, whereas the higher-calorie hindmilk is thicker and creamier, resembling whole milk. If your baby is not gaining weight sufficiently and your health care provider suspects insufficient milk volume or calorie content, an analysis of the fat content of your milk can be performed. This is not, however, routinely done in the evaluation of insufficient milk supply.

Your baby's contentment level during and between feeding is also a guide to whether he is receiving sufficient milk. If you feel that your baby is sucking vigorously, if you hear him swallowing, feel your milk ejection reflex and then see the baby drift contentedly off to sleep, chances are he has gotten enough milk. A baby who awakens frequently during the day and night and does not seem content after a feeding may not be getting enough in volume and/or in calorie content.

12

NIPPLE CARE

Teaching your baby to latch on correctly to your areola is the best preventive medicine for sore nipples. At the first sign of nipple soreness, scrutinize your technique of positioning and latch-on to be sure you are not letting the baby apply most of the pressure to your nipples rather than to the areola. Be especially sure that baby is opening his mouth wide enough and flanging both lips (especially the lower). Be sure your nipples are completely dry at all times when not "in use." Use fresh nursing pads, without plastic liners, to be sure no moisture is in contact with your tender skin. Let your nipples dry thoroughly before you put your bra flap up; it may be necessary to air your nipples for awhile before closing your bra. If you're in a hurry, try using a blow dryer (on low setting and only for a short time) to speed this process.

A pure oil (vegetable or vitamin E capsule, one drop, three times in 24 hours) to which neither mother nor father is allergic, completely massaged into the nipples after nursing, can provide local soothing and healing. The best massage medium is colostrum or breast milk. Do not use oils or creams that need to be washed off before nursing, even if the hospital offers you one. The little bumps on your areola around the nipple are glands that secret a cleansing and lubricating oil to protect the nipples and keep them clean. Avoid using soap on your nipples, since it may encourage dryness and cracking and it removes those natural cleansing and lubricating oils. A pure vegetable oil will absorb into the skin of your areola before your next nursing, so you don't have to wash it off. Careful sunbathing (only for a few minutes) can also speed healing.

If your nipples are getting sore from baby clamping down too hard (review the steps for positioning and latch-on), pull down his lower jaw slightly during sucking and pull him closer into your breast during nursing. Put baby to the side that is least sore first and encourage more frequent, shorter feedings. If baby needs to be pacified and your nipples are wearing out, let him suck on an index finger instead of a pacifier (dads use the pinky finger) in the early weeks to avoid nipple confusion or poor suck patterns. Cut your nails short and get the finger (nail down against the tongue) in as far as you can, about 1½ inches.

Nursing less frequently usually does not help sore nipples, since engorgement may result. A hungrier baby also nurses more intensely, which further aggravates the soreness. Remember not to pull your baby off the nipple at the end of each nursing, but rather break the suction by inserting your finger into the corner of his mouth and gently lifting his lips and gums off the nipple.

In our experience, nipple shields are of little value in the treatment of sore nipples, but a breast shield or breast shell ("sore nipple ring") worn between—not during—nursing sessions may be helpful when nipples are cracked. (See Key 22 on the use of breast shields and for warnings against the use of nipple shields.) If nipple soreness continues, consult your lactation specialist or La Leche League.

13

INCREASING MILK SUPPLY

Most insufficient milk production is the result of improper positioning and latch-on, failure to room-in, and interference with the harmony between mother and baby (giving supplemental bottles, trying to schedule feedings, and being too busy). Go through the following checklist:

- **Avoid supplemental formula** unless medically necessary.
- **Are you too busy?** Temporarily shelve all other commitments that drain your energy away from getting in harmony with your baby, and delegate household responsibilities to other members. Settle your nest a bit if there are too many household distractions that interfere with nursing.
- **Avoid negative advisors** with comments such as, "Are you sure he's getting enough milk?" and "I couldn't breastfeed either. . . ." You don't need discouragement when you're trying to build up your confidence as a new mother. Surround yourself with supportive people. Breastfeeding is a confidence game.
- **Take your baby to bed with you** and nurse and nestle close to each other. Nap nursing and night nursing are powerful stimulators for milk production, since the milk-producing hormones are best secreted while you sleep.
- **Increase the frequency of feedings** to at least one feeding every two to three hours; wake your baby during the day if he sleeps more than three hours. Even a sleepy baby will nestle against your breast and stimulate your milk.

- **Look at, caress, and groom your baby** while nursing. These maternal behaviors stimulate the milk-producing hormones.
- **Sleep when your baby sleeps.** This requires delaying or delegating many of the seemingly pressing household chores. If you are blessed with a baby who nurses frequently, you may think, "I don't get anything done." But you *are* getting something done.
- **Undress your baby during nursing.** If baby is small (under eight pounds), you need to keep a blanket around him that still allows skin-to-skin contact. This will awaken a sleepy baby and stimulate a less enthusiastic nurse.
- **Try switch nursing.** In a traditional method of nursing, you encourage your baby to nurse as long as he wishes on one breast (usually around 10 to 15 minutes) and to complete his feeding on the second breast, reversing the process on the next feeding. For a baby who falls asleep too soon, try switch nursing, also called the "burp-and-switch technique," which operates as follows. Let baby nurse on the first breast until the intensity of his suck and swallow diminishes and his eyes start to close (usually four to five minutes). Remove him from this breast and burp him well; then switch to the next breast until his sucking diminishes again. Stop, burp him a second time, and repeat the entire process back on the first breast, and so on. This burp-and-switch technique encourages a creamier, higher-calorie hindmilk to come into your breast at each feeding. The method operates on the principle that as you are feeding from one breast, the creamier and higher-calorie hindmilk is letting down from the back of the other breast, so that by the time the baby gets to the second breast he gets the more high-powered milk. This fact accounts for the saying, "Babies grow best at the second breast." Breast massage before and during feeding also releases hindmilk.

- **Try double nursing.** This technique of double nursing operates on this same principle of increasing the volume and fat content of your milk. After you nurse your baby and he seems to be content, carry him around in a baby carrier instead of immediately putting him down to sleep. Burp him well and, about 20 minutes later, breastfeed baby a second time. Keeping baby upright for 10 to 20 minutes following a feeding allows the trapped bubble of air to be burped up, leaving room for topping off.
- **Be sure you are able to relax during feeding.** The milk ejection reflex can be inhibited if you are physically or emotionally tense. Use the relaxation techniques you learned in childbirth class, use pillows, have someone rub your back, visualize flowing streams.
- **Eat right** during breastfeeding as you did during pregnancy. See Key 18 for suggestions on nutrition during lactation.
- **Natural herbs to increase your milk supply.** Many herbs and home remedies have been touted to increase milk production, based more on folklore than on real evidence. However, we have found *fenugreek tea* to be very effective. Brew a cup of tea by steeping 1 teaspoon of fenugreek seeds in a cup of boiling water for about 5 minutes, or until the water is nicely colored and scented (the tea has a sweetish flavor reminiscent of maple). I (Martha) have found a few cups of this tea to be very helpful during times when my milk supply seems to be lagging.
- **Don't give up** if your milk supply is still insufficient. See a lactation specialist for more help.

14

AVOIDING AND TREATING ENGORGEMENT

Engorgement—a pronounced **filling** and **swelling** of the breasts that causes them to be very hard and painful, and that makes it difficult for baby to get a good latch-on—is your body's signal that the supply-and-demand mechanism is out of balance. Engorgement is a problem for both mother and baby. For mother, it can be very painful and, if left untreated, it can progress to a debilitating breast infection. The condition is also uncomfortable for baby; if your breasts are engorged the nipple angle flattens, preventing baby from properly latching on. When this happens, your baby sucks your nipples but cannot get enough of the breast in his mouth to compress the milk sinuses. As a result, baby stimulates more milk to enter the breast but is unable to empty it, further aggravating engorgement and setting up a vicious cycle. Baby gets less milk and nurses more frequently; mother gets more engorged and the nursing pair is in trouble. You can prevent engorgement by following the right start tips for breastfeeding: rooming-in, feeding on cue rather than by schedule, and using correct positioning and latch-on technique.

If engorgement occurs while you are still in the hospital, use an electric breast pump to release some of the extra milk in order to soften the areola, so that baby can latch on better and more effectively empty your breasts. Usually the breasts slowly and steadily build up milk in the first week, and baby should empty the breast at the rate the milk appears. Some engorgement is common as your milk appears during the first week, but it should subside with proper positioning and latch-on, frequent nursing and lots of rest. Sometimes mother's milk appears "suddenly" around the third or fourth day, causing mothers to exclaim, "I awakened with these two painful boulders on my chest." Request an electric breast pump immediately to relieve this engorgement before it progresses.

Engorgement at home can be dealt with by using manual expression or a manual pump (see Key 23 on selecting the right breast pump). A warm shower, warm soaking in a basin or applying warm compresses for 10 minutes before expressing or feeding will help trigger your milk ejection reflex so you can let go of some of this overabundance. If your breasts are too engorged for baby to effectively latch on, manually express some milk prior to feeding to soften your areola enough that your baby can grasp the areola and not only the nipple. If engorgement is extremely painful, use continuous ice packs between feedings to alleviate the pain. This will also reduce the swelling, allowing your milk to flow. Tylenol for pain and a well-fitting bra for support are also helpful; so is rest. Above all, don't stop nursing! The breasts must be emptied.

Engorgement in later weeks of breastfeeding is often due to an upset in the baby's or the family's routine—too many visitors, missed feedings, too many outside activities, use of supplemental formulas, anything that throws the "timer" out of balance. If you have enjoyed weeks or months of uncomplicated breastfeeding and suddenly you are becoming engorged, take inventory of your feeding techniques. This is usually a signal that your nest or your schedule is too busy. Listen to your body; it's trying to tell you something.

15

WHAT TO WEAR

Wearing comfortable and fashionable clothing during breastfeeding will help you better enjoy this style of feeding your baby.

Selecting the right bra. Nursing bras are especially designed with a flap on the cup that is opened for feedings. During pregnancy, purchase a bra that is one numerical size larger *and* one cup size larger than you usually wear. Before baby is born, purchase one or two bras that are even an additional size larger, allowing for breast enlargement when your milk appears. After the second week, when your milk is established and your breasts are at their maximum size but no longer swollen, purchase two or three bras of the appropriate size. Above all, avoid tight-fitting bras, as they encourage breast infections.

In selecting a nursing bra, look for the following: Avoid bras with underwires, since these wires may compress the breast, leading to infection. The bra cup should be 100 percent cotton, and should never contain a plastic liner (which does not allow the breast to breathe). Take great care to select a bra that fastens and unfastens easily with one hand so that you don't have to put the baby down when you open or close the cup. Nursing bras that have a row of hooks down the front are usually unsatisfactory. Those with a hook at the top of each cup offer more support and easier access, letting you uncover one breast at a time. The cup of the bra should support the entire lower half of the breast in a natural position when the flap is down. You will need at least three nursing bras, one on you, one in the laundry, and one hanging up to dry. To absorb leaking milk, you can use cotton or disposable nursing pads (again, without plastic liners). Or you can use a folded all-cotton handkerchief in each cup of your bra, or cut out four-inch circles from all-cotton diapers. Avoid synthetic fabrics and no-iron finishes, as these are not absorbent. Be sure to change the breast pads often enough to keep your breasts dry. Nursing bras can be purchased from maternity shops and department stores, or through La Leche League and catalogs.

Nursing fashions. It is very common for a new mother to come into our office for her first baby's checkup and to feel very awkward trying to breastfeed in a one-piece dress. I have seen mothers in this type of outfit absolutely go into contortions trying to disrobe quickly to comfort their screaming babies. They sometimes actually forget where they are because of the overwhelming maternal urge to get the breast out as quickly as possible and silence the crying baby. Proper nursing fashions allow discreet breastfeeding.

Specially designed *nursing blouses* have slits with Velcro fasteners over each breast that are easily opened to make your breast accessible for quick and easy nursing. Avoid full slips; half slips are much more practical. Most one-piece dresses are not conducive to convenient and discreet breastfeeding, but you can order them with specially designed nursing flaps and slips out of maternity fashion catalogs. Two-piece outfits and warmup suits are ideal. The blouse or sweater should be loose and easily lifted from the waist for nursing, with baby covering any bare midriff.

Wear blouses that button in the front and remember to unbutton the blouse from the bottom up, using the unbuttoned flap of the blouse to cover baby for inconspicuous nursing.

Pullover sweaters are particularly easy for nursing. Shawls and scarves are attractive and practical apparel for covering baby during discreet breastfeeding; they accent the limited designs available in nursing dresses. Choose prints and colors that won't show any milk that might leak through; avoid white, pale colors, and clinging materials. Don't try to squeeze into your pre-pregnancy clothes too soon. Many mothers find that they will not be able to wear their entire pre-pregnancy wardrobe until nine months after birth. Tight blouses rub against your nipples, are uncomfortable, and can trigger a milk ejection reflex at the most inconvenient time.

If you are particularly sensitive about nursing in public, take great care in choosing your breastfeeding wardrobe and practice breastfeeding in front of a mirror until you are comfortable with all the motions and are able to feed discreetly. Think of how you can tuck your baby's face inside rather than bring your breast out.

One of the most recent innovations in nursing fashions is the use of baby carriers designed for nursing. Mothers the world over fabricate a sling-type carrier as an extension of their native dress or using the same material and design as their dress. Baby is worn in the sling very near mother's breast. During breastfeeding mother simply lifts part of the sling over baby's head and offers her breast. The nursing pair can nurse anywhere comfortably and inconspicuously. Your nursing wardrobe should include:

- Nursing bras—at least three
- Breast pads
- Nursing blouses and dresses
- A baby sling

16

RELAXING DURING BREASTFEEDING

At times motherhood can be tension-producing and you may find yourself unable to relax during feedings. Tension and stress can actually inhibit your milk ejection reflex (MER). If your baby picks up on this you may also have a tense, anxious baby, especially if the inhibited MER results in a lessened milk flow.

Within each breastfeeding mother exists a self-inducing relaxation system resulting from the hormone prolactin. Any activity that increases a breastfeeding mother's prolactin will help her relax. Before you actually being to breastfeed, set yourself up for all those womanly activities that increase your prolactin. *Think baby.* Imagine yourself breastfeeding. Imagine pictures of your baby, the facial expressions you enjoy most, the movements you enjoy most. All these images of your baby get the relaxing hormones flowing. If you are not in the same room with your baby (e.g., if he is asleep and you are working somewhere else in the house), besides imaging-ing your baby, look at appealing pictures of him.

Massage your baby. Stroke and cuddle him using a lot of skin-to-skin contact, a custom called grooming. This activity will also increase your prolactin. Minimize distractions during breastfeeding. Take the phone off the hook; nurse in a quiet room. Minimize all those outside disturbances that will distract you from breastfeeding your baby.

Eat a healthful snack and drink extra water or juice prior to nursing. A warm bath, a hot shower or a brief nap before a feeding is also good therapy for a relaxed nursing experience. The breathing exercises and relaxation techniques you learn during childbirth class can be useful if you are particularly tense prior to breastfeeding. Play some soothing music prior to and during your breastfeeding. Have someone stand behind you and massage your neck, shoulders and upper back, especially along the upper spine to get specific release for the area of tension that can inhibit your MER. If you are alone you can do this yourself by rubbing your back up against the corner of a wall or doorway.

Prepare a nursing station. Choose your favorite room in the house, usually one that is well lighted, airy, pleasant, but not too distracting. The station contains your favorite chair (preferably a rocking chair with arms at a comfortable height to support your arms while holding baby), plenty of pillows, a footstool (see Key 22 for breastfeeding aids), soothing music, a relaxing book, extra juice or water for you as you become thirsty, and a tray full of nutritious nibbles right next to your chair.

The nursing station concept works well while breastfeeding a baby in addition to caring for a busy toddler—a combination that prevents many breastfeeding mothers from relaxing. If your toddler becomes disruptive as soon as you begin to breastfeed your baby, causing you to become tense, try the following: Put some nutritious snacks on the nursing station table for your toddler. Include a basket of your toddler's favorite toys right next to the rocking chair, and a couple of your toddler's favorite books or tapes. Reserve these books, toys, and activities only for nursing time so that your toddler learns that nursing time for baby is also a special time for him. As your new baby is nestled in one arm and nursing, you then have another arm (and a couple of feet) free to play with your toddler. If your toddler wants to climb into the chair with you, try using a mat on the floor as your place to sit (supported with pillows). This could even be in his room so you can close the door, limiting the area he can get into. It's hard to relax if you know the older one is off in another room getting into mischief.

If you try the nursing station idea, you will notice that instead of your toddler clicking into undesirable behavior as soon as he sees you sit down to nurse, he may start enjoying the feeling that now mom does special things with me that she does not do at any other time. And hopefully you will have some one-on-one time each day with your toddler when baby is sleeping. This one-on-one time can then extend into a sleeping time for all three of you. Now *that's* relaxing.

Try breastfeeding in the bathtub. One of the best ways to relax prior to and during breastfeeding is to sit in a warm bath with the water level just below your breasts. Breastfeed baby (who is also about half-immersed in warm water) as you recline in the tub. It is usually safer to have someone else hand you the baby after you position yourself in the tub, or to place baby on a towel next to the tub till you get yourself settled. Trying to step into a filled tub while holding the baby poses the risk of slipping.

Relaxing during breastfeeding is self-perpetuating. Getting yourself relaxed to enjoy a successful breastfeeding stimulates hormones that cause you to relax still more, and the cycle continues. As one busy mother put it, "Whenever I'm tense, I sit down and nurse. My baby relaxes me."

17

DOES BABY NEED EXTRA WATER, VITAMINS OR IRON?

Water. Breastfed babies do not need extra water, but formula-fed babies do. Breast milk is very high in water content, whereas formula is more concentrated and extra water is needed to make it easier for baby's immature kidneys to process it. Breastfeeding specialists generally discourage extra water, not because of the water itself, but because of the possibility of nipple confusion if babies are given water in a bottle.

Vitamin supplements. Though premature infants should receive iron and vitamin supplements, a healthy, full-term baby who is getting enough breast milk does not need them. Human milk contains adequate quantities of all essential vitamins. Some nutritionists believe that breast milk may be deficient in vitamin D, but it does not seem possible that a milk that has been adapted for survival of the species should be deficient in any nutrient. I suspect that although the quantity of vitamin D in human milk may seem low on paper, its biological activity (the amount that is actually absorbed and utilized) is adequate to meet the infant's needs as long as the infant is exposed to sunlight. Vitamin D is derived from two sources: the exposure of the skin to sunlight (this converts compounds within the skin to vitamin D), and the ingestion of vitamin D-enriched from certain foods. If your diet is for some reason low in vitamin D, or if you live in an area where exposure to sunlight is limited, especially during the winter months, your doctor may recommend vitamin D supplements.

Iron supplements. Older medical books recommend giving iron supplements to breastfeeding babies because analysis of breast milk showed it to be low in iron. New techniques in measuring iron have revealed that breastfed infants do not need supplements. While the iron content of breast milk is "low," the iron is biologically very active. What matters is not how much iron the milk contains, but how much gets into the baby's bloodstream. It may well be that only 10 percent of the iron added to formulas and cereals is absorbed by the baby; of the iron in breast milk, 50 to 75 percent is absorbed. Unless you are so advised by your doctor or your baby's hemoglobin level is low, iron supplements are not needed.

Whether breastfed infants should have fluoride supplements is still controversial. Human milk, like cow's milk, contains very little fluoride, irrespective of the fluoride content of the water supply. Studies show that the frequency of dental caries in breastfed, non-fluoride-supplemented infants is identical to that of infants who are fed formula diluted with naturally fluoridated water. Studies in communities with fluoridated water supplies suggest that fluoride obtained after the age of six to eight months is sufficient to decrease the number of caries in the permanent teeth. The Committee on Nutrition of the American Academy of Pediatrics recommends that fluoride supplements be given to both breast and formula-fed infants beginning at age two weeks in areas where the water is not adequately fluoridated. It is wise to check with your pediatric dentist about the fluoride content in your water and when and if a fluoride supplement should be given to your baby. Researchers have concluded that fluoride ingested by the mother does not reach the baby through her milk.

18

EATING RIGHT AND STAYING TRIM

As you were "eating for two" during your pregnancy, you are also eating for two during lactation. Consider the following tips for healthy eating for you and your baby during breastfeeding.

- Most breastfeeding mothers require an extra 500 to 600 calories per day to provide adequate nutrition for themselves and their babies. This figure is simply an average. If you were overweight prior to or during your pregnancy, you may require fewer calories as the excess fat stores in your body are gradually used up. If you were underweight you may require more. It is interesting that undernutrition during lactation will affect mother more than baby. This is why babies are often called "the perfect parasite," meaning that if there is not enough nutrition to go around, baby will get it and mother will suffer (the adage is more true during pregnancy, however, than during lactation). Both mother and baby will suffer if mother is extremely malnourished, but it takes more than a slight degree of undernutrition to harm the quality and quantity of your breast milk.
- Eat nutrient-dense foods such as vegetables—foods that have a lot of nutrition for each calorie. Avoid "empty calories," (sweets, desserts, and most snack foods). For balanced nutrition stress the four basic food groups:
  - Protein foods: poultry, fish, lean meat, eggs, legumes
  - Dairy products: yogurt, cheese, milk

- Grains and cereals: bread, pasta, rice
- Fruits and vegetables

It is wise to have three to four servings of each of these food groups each day. Most calories should come in the form of complex carbohydrates (vegetables, fruits and grains). Sugars, or simple carbohydrates, cause a sudden rise and a rapid fall in blood sugar, along with swings in mood and energy level. Complex carbohydrates contain the types of "good sugars" that are more slowly digested and utilized in your body. Because they take longer to digest, they do not stimulate a craving for more sugars and do not cause mood swings. A balanced diet should provide 50 to 55 percent of your calories in the form of carbohydrates (mostly the complex type), 30 percent fat and 15 to 20 percent protein.

- **Calcium** is very important during pregnancy and lactation. Calcium is important to baby because of his rapidly growing bones. You don't have to drink milk to make milk—cows don't! If you are allergic to milk, if you don't like milk or if you're lactose intolerant, you can get all the calcium you need from calcium-rich nondairy foods: sardines, broccoli, soybeans, salmon, tofu, collards, kale, watercress, okra, grains, and dried beans. If you dislike milk, yogurt and cheese are good dairy sources of calcium.
- **Iron** is vital to the pregnant and lactating mother. Iron-rich foods are mainly organ meats (liver, kidney and heart), fish, poultry, and iron-fortified cereals. While vegetables contain some iron, they are not a good source of the nutrient for humans. Eating vitamin C–rich foods along with iron-rich foods (combinations like orange juice and iron-fortified cereal, or meatballs with tomato sauce) improves absorption of the iron. Egg yolk has a high iron content but not easily absorbed.

Egg whites are a very good source of protein for the lactating mother; an egg a day is recommended. If you are prone to cholesterol problems or have a family history of high cholesterol, it is wise not to exceed three egg yolks per week, but there is no restriction on egg whites.

- **Vitamin supplements.** Most nutritionists recommend continuing your prenatal vitamin supplements during lactation. Exposure to sunlight is a ready source of additional vitamin D. If your baby is fussy, you may need to change to a different brand of vitamin supplement. We have found that several common prescription brands of prenatal vitamins contain an iron salt that seems to cause colic in some babies. Switching to an over-the-counter healthfood store brand cured the problem.
- **Vegetarian diets** during lactation should be followed only in consultation with a nutritionist. It is important to combine the right vegetable proteins, eat iron-containing foods and perhaps supplement the strict vegetarian diet with eggs and dairy products.
- **Extra fluids** are very necessary during breastfeeding. You will require at least six to eight glasses of liquid a day; it is wise to have a glass of water or juice shortly before each breastfeeding. As a rule of thumb, drink as your thirst guides you plus a glass or two more each day. Avoid caffeine-containing coffee and tea and alcoholic beverages; these may have a diuretic effect, causing you to lose valuable fluids and minerals. Frequent intake of water, soups, and juice should be part of your daily routine.

As a general rule you can eat anything during breastfeeding, but there is a wide range of infant food intolerances. Here are a few foods that are commonly troublesome.

Foods to avoid while breastfeeding: Caffeine-containing foods and drinks (coffee, tea, cola and chocolate) in excess may cause colicky symptoms in baby. While it is difficult to prove this scientifically, many mothers have reported that gassy foods, such as broccoli, cabbage, onion, Brussels sprouts, cauliflower, and green peppers, especially in the raw state, cause their babies to be gassy. Dairy products taken by the breastfeeding mother have been reported to cause colic in susceptible babies. Less commonly, wheat, eggs, corn, shellfish, nuts may also upset the baby.

It is estimated that it takes four to six hours for the food you eat to reach your milk. Some foods, among them spices and garlic, may cause an unpleasant taste in the milk. If your baby goes through an unexplained colicky period or refuses to nurse, taste your milk to detect any changed or unpleasant flavor; also examine your diet.

To minimize the risk of environmental pollutants entering your milk, avoid fish from waters known to be contaminated; peel and thoroughly wash fresh fruits and vegetables. Cut away the fatty portions of meat, poultry, and fish, since chemicals tend to be concentrated in fat.

Foods that make milk. To our knowledge, no foods have been proven to make milk; most "remedies" are a matter of folklore. Most lactation specialists believe that foods and drinks touted to increase milk supply have a mainly psychological benefit; the mother thinks her milk will be better, so she relaxes more and the milk becomes better because of her relaxation, not because of the particular food. There may, however, be an exception: from personal experience we have found fenugreek tea to be a helpful stimulant to milk production.

Losing weight during lactation. A safe rule of thumb is a maximum weight loss of no more than one pound per week during lactation, but even safer might be a figure of 2½ pounds per month. The safe limit of weight loss will be greater if you were overweight to begin with, less if you were underweight. A breastfeeding mother at her ideal weight can eat 500 extra nutritious calories per day without abnormal weight gain. This figure depends on your body type and on whether you were over- or underweight to begin with.

If you are gaining weight during breastfeeding you are probably eating too much; if you are losing more than one pound a week (preferably 2½ pounds a month) you are probably eating too little. Avoid crash diets during lactation; the key is to lose weight *gradually.* Nutritionists think that diets under 2,000 nutritious calories a day cannot supply enough calories for the health and well-being of mother and baby.

A gradual weight loss is also safer because of the lessened chance of environmental pollutants getting into the bloodstream. Chemicals such as pesticides and toxic metals in freshwater fish are concentrated in the body fat. A rapid reduction in body fat (greater than one pound per week) may cause too many of these chemicals to be released into the mother's bloodstream and thus into her baby. Again, gradual is the key to safe weight loss.

Exercise is the safest way to lose weight during lactation because you wish to lose excess fat, not lean body mass (muscle and bone tissue). Crash diets of insufficient nutrient-dense foods are likely to diminish lean body mass, whereas exercise only burns off excess fat.

Consider these exercise tips: Choose an activity you enjoy; you are more likely to stick with it. A very comfortable exercise for mother (and baby) is to put the baby in a sling and take at least a one-hour walk every day. Walking briskly while carrying baby for one hour will burn off an average of 400 calories. This exercise plus one less chocolate chip cookie or its equivalent in junk food will burn off around a pound a week (a deficit of 500 calories a day or 3,500 calories per week will result in one-pound weight loss). Exercise after breastfeeding is usually most comfortable, since your breasts are less full and cumbersome. Be sure to wear a good supportive bra during vigorous exercise. Soft breast pads are also necessary to prevent friction on your nipples.

The following weight-control program is one we have used successfully in our breastfeeding center.

1. Set a safe and realistic goal (average 2½ pounds per month—more if overweight, less if underweight to begin with).
2. Set what you feel is an optimal number of calories for your health and well-being (average around 2,000 **nutritious** calories a day, balanced among the four basic food groups).
3. Exercise one hour per day—an activity that you enjoy and preferably one that you can do with your baby.
4. Chart your progress. If you are still gaining weight while following this program, you are probably eating too much. If you are losing weight according to your goal and still feeling good, then you have arrived at the optimum number of calories you can consume.

We have noted that some mothers cannot do aerobics more than once or twice a week. Their babies become fussy, usually because the milk supply drops due to the mother's energy expenditure. There have even been reports of the taste of the milk being affected by too much vigorous exercise. Also, upper-body exertion of any kind, such as jumping rope, pushing a lawn mower, or performing upper arm exercises, can occasionally bring about mastitis.

19

PREVENTING AND TREATING BREAST INFECTIONS

A breast infection (the medical term is mastitis) usually results from engorgement not having been recognized and treated early enough. A basic principle of human biology is that fluid that is stuck anywhere in the body will eventually get infected. Milk that becomes stagnant in the breasts provides an excellent medium for the growth of bacteria. This is why breastfeeding consultants stress the importance of keeping the milk flowing, emptying the breasts as much as possible through frequent feedings. Milk that sits too long within the breast, either from going too long without a feeding or from a clogged duct, is a setup for infection. To prevent a breast infection, first follow all the steps for preventing breast engorgement (see Key 14).

Recognizing if you have breast infection. Symptoms of mastitis very much resemble the flu: generalized fatigue, muscle aches, fever, and chills. It is a medical truism that a breastfeeding mother with "flu" has mastitis until proven otherwise. The involved area of the breast may show the four typical signs of infection: it is reddened, hot, tender, and swollen. Sometimes breast infection may begin only with a small, square-inch area of tenderness to the touch and generalized flulike symptoms. More often than not, the infection occurs only in one breast and usually in the outer half of the breast.

When does engorgement or a clogged duct become a breast infection? Sometimes a breast may be painfully engorged, a mother may be achy and flulike and even have a low-grade fever, but infection has not yet set in. After using all the treatments outlined for engorgement (see Key 14), if fever, chills, and breast tenderness are worsening—not to mention overall feeling of unwellness—consider this a breast infection rather than only engorgement.

Nearly all breast infections begin with breast engorgement or an area of engorgement, but not all engorgement progresses to an infection. A plugged milk duct is a lumpy area in the breast that is reddened and painful to the touch but initially without any associated symptoms of fever and chills. Applying moist heat (a hot, wet towel or a jet of hot water in the shower) and emptying your breast frequently and completely should unclog the duct and cause the lump to subside. If the lump progresses rapidly in size and tenderness and is accompanied by flulike symptoms, consider it a breast infection. The most severe type of infection occurs when a localized area of tenderness begins developing a boillike appearance, becoming exquisitely tender, red and hot and accompanied with fever and chills. This may signify an underlying breast abscess.

To treat a breast infection, go through these steps.

- Review the correct latch-on and positioning and proper breastfeeding techniques. Are you missing too many feedings? Is baby sleeping through feedings? Is there stress in the household? Are you being overworked? In other words, is there anything going on within your breastfeeding environment that interferes with the law of supply and demand, or that causes the milk not to flow freely and frequently?
- Try traditional self-help remedies, just as you would with the flu: bed rest, lots of fluids, and pain medications that

are safe to take while breastfeeding (see Key 31 for safe medications).

- Above all, don't stop nursing, despite any erroneous advice you may receive to the contrary. Your breast needs to empty for the infection to be relieved (though strictly speaking, breasts never *completely* empty). If your infected breast is too tender and the infection is severe, breastfeed your baby on the non-infected breast but express or pump the infected breast. Apply moist heat by immersing the infected breast into comfortably warm water, standing in a hot shower with a jet of warm water on your breast, or placing a hot compress on the infected area. Follow this with proper breast pressure massage (starting at the chest wall and working down toward the nipple) to empty the breast. Get the milk out any way you can.
- Some breastfeeding consultants even recommend offering the sore breast first in order to more completely empty it. This is possible if the infection and soreness is mild. Manually express right before offering the sore breast so as to soften the areola, minimize engorgement and make latch-on more comfortable and effective.
- A position that may seem unusual but which is extremely effective in emptying the breast is the "all fours" posture which uses the effect of gravity plus the efficient sucking of the baby. After applying moist heat, place your baby on the bed and position yourself above him, allowing your breast to hang straight down. Let baby suck actively for as long as possible. If baby is not able, perhaps your husband would be willing, or a third choice would be to use a breast pump in this position.
- Call your doctor for an appropriate antibiotic and pain-relieving medication that is safe to take while breastfeeding. The three classes of antibiotics that are safe to take during breastfeeding are penicillin, cephalosporin and erythro-

mycin. Usually a broad-spectrum antibiotic is given and is effective against the two most common organisms, staphylococcus and streptococcus.

- Wear a supporting bra but be sure it is not too tight.
- Change your baby's position with every feeding so that the pressure of sucking will be applied to different places on the breast and exert pressure on different ducts. Sleep on your back or side without putting pressure on the involved breast.
- Unless your doctor advises otherwise, or the infection is severe, it is all right for the baby to feed from the infected breast. Occasionally baby may refuse this breast because of the salty taste of the milk. In this case let him nurse on the other breast and express the milk from the infected side manually or with a breast pump.

Properly treated, the flulike symptoms accompanying a breast infection should lessen within 24 to 48 hours, with gradual recovery over the next week. Be sure to finish *all* of the antibiotic. If you have repeated breast infections, review your methods of latch-on, the frequency of feedings, and the fit of your bra, and do what you can to make your environment less stressful and busy. It would be wise to seek help from a lactation consultant or physician if you are prone to repeated breast infections.

20

SUPPLEMENTING THE BREASTFEEDING BABY

Unless you are advised otherwise for a medical reason, breastfeeding babies do not need supplemental bottles of formula or water. Milk production works on the principle of supply and demand—the more your infant nurses properly, the more milk you will produce until a balance is achieved. Breastfeeding problems occur when this balance is upset. It is the frequency of nursing and the duration of feedings that stimulate the milk-producing glands. Supplemental bottles throw nursing harmony out of balance. Babies who are given supplemental bottles may nurse less frequently, causing painful engorgement of the breast and eventually a decrease in milk supply. Supplemental feedings should be avoided and nursing schedules should be set by baby's internal clock to maintain the desired balance between milk production and demand.

Sucking on artificial nipples can lead to nipple confusion, which will throw mother and baby off harmony just at the time when baby is learning how to suck from the breast and mother and baby are attempting to get in sync with each other. When breast and bottle are both offered, especially in the early weeks, nipple confusion may occur; it is less of a problem later on. During this important time of behavior patterning, the baby can imprint incorrectly since the technique for sucking on a rubber nipple is different from that of sucking at the breast. For example, when a baby sucks from a rubber nipple, milk flow begins immediately and the entire suck-swallow mechanism of tongue and jaw coordination is different. At mother's breast he must work for 30 to 60 seconds or more before his efforts are rewarded, and the suck-swallow mechanism is not the same as with the bottle. A newborn may become understandably confused when his learned behavior pattern is not reinforced as anticipated, i.e., he expects the breast and gets the bottle.

Not all babies experience nipple confusion. Quite often a baby can be given supplemental bottles in the early weeks for a medical reason and then settle down to a total and comfortable breastfeeding experience. The problem is that early on we don't know which babies are going to be prone to nipple confusion and which are not. Therefore, it is wise to avoid artificial nipples unless absolutely necessary. It is not so much the supplemental formula that interferes with breastfeeding (although this too can upset the law of supply and demand), it is how the formula is given that leads to nipple confusion.

If baby does need a supplement for medical reasons, e.g. prematurity, temporary poor suck, etc., the combination of syringe feedings and finger sucking (finger feeding) is a good alternative. In this method, father, mother, or nurse uses a finger (inserted nail down about 1½ inches), for the baby to suck on. During the finger sucking, a syringe is used (periodontal syringes [with a curved tip], available from a dental supply house, work well). Formula or preferably pumped breast milk is used in the syringe; the tip is inserted just inside the corner of the baby's mouth. As baby is sucking on the finger, milk is gently squirted at a rate easily swallowed.

Another alternative to supplemental bottles is the use of a **Supplemental Nutrition System** (SNS). This ingenious little device consists of a flexible plastic bottle that hangs from mother's neck and rests between her breasts. Two tiny polyethylene tubings come from a bottle and rest alongside mother's nipple, taped in place along the breast. Pumped breast milk or formula is placed in the bottle. When baby sucks from mother's nipple he also sucks on the tubing and gets milk from the bottle. Baby thinks this milk is coming from mother. The use of the syringe-finger feeding and SNS gives babies the supplement they need without causing nipple confusion by sucking on an artificial nipple.

If mothers choose to breastfeed part-time and supplemental bottles are necessary (see Key 26 on breastfeeding and working), consider the following.

1. Wait several weeks till your breastfeeding relationship is well established.
2. Try to use supplements when your milk supply is lowest, usually at the end of the day.
3. Use the same nurturing technique during bottle-feeding as you would during breastfeeding: hold your baby toward you, bottle up against your breast with a lot of skin-to-skin and eye-to-eye contact, and relate to your baby during the bottle feeding. Remember, there should always be a relating person at both ends of a breast or a bottle.

21

SEXUALITY DURING BREASTFEEDING

Yes, there is sex after childbirth! After giving birth and during breastfeeding, a new mother will undergo normal emotional and physiological changes in her sexuality. Understanding why these changes occur and how to keep the sexual fires burning during lactation is a normal part of new parents' maturity.

A season of the marriage. Prior to birth a woman's sexual hormones are higher than her maternal hormones. After birth and during lactation the reverse occurs. This increase of maternal over sexual hormones may dominate until weaning. A woman's desire to take care of her baby may take priority over her desire for sexual intimacy with her husband. This shift seems to be part of the normal design for the survival of the species.

Fatigue is another reason for a woman's diminishing sexual interest during breastfeeding. New mothers often feel so drained by the constant demands of the baby that they have little energy left over for sex. Mothers whom we have interviewed on this topic feel "all used up."

Sexual responsiveness after birth and during lactation varies tremendously among women. Some women actually experience a heightened sexual responsiveness during breastfeeding. Others experience highs and lows of sexual interest during breastfeeding, one week feeling very sexually responsive and the next week feeling very uninterested.

Expect a few normal bodily nuisances to occur during lovemaking and breastfeeding, which a bit of understanding and humor will overcome. The hormones that stimulate a milk ejection reflex are also high at the time of orgasm, causing milk to spray out just then. It is not unusual for a baby to awaken right in the middle of lovemaking, even if baby is in another room. Also, because the hormone estrogen is lower when breastfeeding, vaginal dryness may be experienced. This is normal after childbirth and during lactation, and the use of water-soluble lubricants should alleviate the problem. If intercourse is painful, you should consult your obstetrician.

Husbands often have trouble understanding the sexual changes in their wives after childbirth. Although your hormones change, your husband's do not. Husbands often complain that sex is no longer spontaneous; it has to be planned and scheduled to fit in with the competing demands of another individual in the family. Consider the following ideas for achieving sexual harmony after birth.

Communicate your needs and feelings. Talk to your husband about your disinterest. Explain the hormonal changes we described earlier so he can understand that you are feeling the way you do because you are designed that way, not because he has done anything to turn you off. Be sure he understands how tired you are. Your husband needs to know that it is *not his fault*, that sex is not the same after childbirth as it was before. Tell your husband what you need. He may be feeling that you no longer want him because the baby has taken his place. Let your husband know that you still need him and that you need and want to be held and touched.

Be responsive. The chief complaint we receive from frustrated fathers is, "She doesn't respond to me." When asked about this, mothers often reply, "I'm too tired" or "I need my sleep more than he needs sex" or "My baby needs me so much that I want to save up my energy for her." Sometimes mothers may seem to be physically with their husband but mentally with their babies, and fathers can sense this detachment. Mothers often have difficulty releasing themselves from the obligations of one role and giving themselves permission to experience the joys of another. Release, respond, and enjoy your husband. For a mother-baby attachment to work in the way it was designed to work, it must be practiced in the structure of a stable and fulfilled marriage. In the attachment style of parenting, the whole family works together—mother-baby, father-baby, and husband-wife. Avoid the "but my baby needs me" syndrome. You should not make an either-or choice among these relationships. You need to work at all of them because they complement each other.

22

HELPFUL BREASTFEEDING AIDS

There once was a time when a baby, a breast and a supportive environment were all that was needed to successfully breastfeed. Because more and more women are now breastfeeding in a variety of medical circumstances and lifestyles, a variety of ingenious aids and resources is now available to make breastfeeding more successful and enjoyable.

Breast shields (also called breast shells and milk cups) are round plastic two-part cups. The outer part is round, like the contour of the breast, and contains a small air hole. (The Medela Breast Shell has multiple air holes to maximize ventilation.) The inner part has a doughnutlike hole in the center to fit over mother's nipple. The parts are interlocking. Breast shields are used in the following circumstances:

- Prenatally for inverted nipples. Wearing the breast shield as much as possible in the last trimester of pregnancy encourages inverted nipples to protrude.
- For inverted nipples postpartum, breast shields can be worn as much as possible between feedings to stimulate nipple protrusion.
- For sore nipples. To keep the bra and clothing from rubbing on the nipples, to keep the nipples dry and to allow air to get to the nipples.

Lactation consultants do not recommend using the milk that has leaked into a breast shield. Breast shields, which are very useful breastfeeding aids, should not be confused with nipple shields, which are not recommended for use without professional supervision. Breast shields and their indications and directions for use are available from your local lactation consultant and La Leche League.

Nipple shields are rubber or silicone nipple shapes that fit over the nipple and areola, forming a vacuum against mother's skin and protecting the nipple. Nipple shields are sometimes recommended to protect sore or cracked nipples during the healing process. They should be used only in extreme circumstances, where mother's nipples have been severely damaged by improper sucking techniques. Most lactation consultants do not recommend the use of nipple shields at all. It is better to focus on correcting the latch-on for the baby than to rely on nipple shields. Used as a last resort, nipple shields may enable a mother to continue who might otherwise feel forced to quit breastfeeding because of severely sore or cracked nipples. They are for short-term use, and only with the close supervision of a lactation specialist. They can actually make the trauma worse if no one is helping to correct the latch-on, and they nearly always result in a drop in milk supply since nipple stimulation is decreased.

Lubricants that moisturize or soften the nipple. Glands within the areola secret natural lubricants and keep the nipple area soft so that artificial lubricants are necessary only if natural lactation has been disturbed (usually by excessive washing with soap). Most lactation specialists find proper positioning and latch-on employing good hygiene, and avoiding soap make artificial lubricants unnecessary. Lubricants may be used with particularly sore, dry and cracked nipples. Those most often recommended by lactation consultants are vitamin E oil (only one drop from the capsule, massaged into the nipple and areola), pure vegetable oil (something you are not allergic to), and anhydrous lanolin (this should be avoided by those allergic to wool). Massage the lubricant gently and sparingly into the sore area of the nipple; avoid excessive amounts on the end of the nipple to avoid clogging the opening. The massaging action increases circulation, which aids healing. Apply the lubricant immediately after nursing and it should be absorbed before the next breastfeeding. Avoid any cream that must be removed before nursing; the very act of wiping it off irritates the nipples. Also avoid any lubricant with a petroleum base, since this prevents the skin from breathing. If you have a history of skin allergies, avoid products containing peanut oil or lanolin. At this writing, most of the breast creams given to mothers in the hospital are either ineffective or potentially harmful and should not be used. Colostrum or breast milk massaged into the nipple and areola is still the best lubricant.

Breast pads are disposable or washable cotton cloth pads that are worn inside the bra to absorb leaking milk. These are commercially available or can be made from cotton handkerchiefs, diapers or sanitary pads. Avoid synthetic fabrics and plastic-lined pads, which cut off air circulation, retain moisture and encourage the growth of bacteria. Pads should be changed frequently after leaking. If the pad sticks to the nipple, moisten it with warm water before peeling it off.

Supplementers (also called supplemental nutrition system or SNS)—see Key 20. These are available from the Medela Company or from La Leche.

A footstool lifts a mother's lap to the correct and most comfortable height for breastfeeding. It eliminates stress on a mother's back, legs, shoulders and arms. The Nursing Stool is especially designed for the breastfeeding mother. It is available from the Medela Company or from La Leche League.

Syringes are helpful to supplement the lazy nurser in lieu of giving supplemental bottles. In our breastfeeding center we use a periodontal syringe, which has a long, curved tip from which supplemental milk (either pumped breast milk or formula) is syringed into the baby's mouth during breastfeeding—or during finger feeding if baby has trouble at the breast.

A baby sling makes life easier and breastfeeding more enjoyable for both mother and baby. The sling-type carrier is much more practical for the breastfeeding pair than either a front, hip, or backpack. A sling allows baby to breastfeed discreetly in public and can be used in a variety of feeding positions. We recommend The Original Baby Sling, and available at nearly all major department stores and baby equipment chains. This sling has been especially designed with the breastfeeding mother and infant in mind.

The above breastfeeding aids are all available by calling your local lactation consultant or La Leche League. See Resources list on page 167.

23

SELECTING THE RIGHT BREAST PUMP

Breast pumps are convenient (and sometimes necessary) breastfeeding aids for expressing milk to relieve engorgement, collecting milk while at work and during medical circumstances when baby or mother is temporarily unable to breastfeed.

Babies suck at the breast in a regular, rhythmic pattern; while no two patterns are identical, there are some significant common characteristics. The breastfeeding cycle consists of three phases: suction, release, relaxation. The entire cycle is completed in approximately one second. This natural, rapid action provides the stimulation necessary for adequate milk flow. It is important to select a breast pump that duplicates this natural breastfeeding pattern as closely as possible, to achieve safe, natural and efficient emptying of the breast. A common misconception among new mothers is that increased vacuum on the breast increases milk flow. Studies indicate, however, that babies breastfeed in bursts and pauses, with a rapid series of quick sucks rather than long, hard pulls. It is the repeated stimulation—not high vacuum—which induces and increases lactation. With some pumps the mother is able to regulate vacuum levels and speed to adjust for individual nipple comfort. Choose a pump that is comfortable for you.

Here are some additional criteria for choosing the right breast pump:

Effectiveness: The pump should efficiently empty the breast (but no pumps will be as efficient as baby).

Safety: The pump should be easy to clean, so that milk residue does not accumulate in the pump mechanism and attract bacteria.

Portability: Be sure your pump is easy to carry to and from work in your purse or in a diaper bag.

Gentleness: The tissues of your breast should not be traumatized by the pump; the process of pumping should not hurt. Avoid pumps with rough edges or uncomfortable suction.

Flexibility: Be sure the pump has two sizes of nipple adapters.

Cost: Varies tremendously, with simple plastic hand pumps being the least expensive and battery-operated and electric pumps the most expensive (the latter are usually rented rather than purchased).

There are basically two types of pumps: Hand and electric. The two general types of hand pumps are cylindrical and bulb-type.

The cylindrical pump is the most popular. It is a very simple design that is easy to clean, transport and operate. It is effective and most mothers do not find it uncomfortable. The pump consists of two cylindrical plastic tubes that fit inside each other and create a vacuum when one cylinder is moved up and down like a piston. Milk is collected into one of the cylinders, which can also be used as a container to store the milk or fitted with a nipple and used as a feeding bottle.

The hand pump that we have used in our breastfeeding

center is the manual/electric pump by Medela. This pump has the advantage of an automatic pressure release that prevents the damage of breast tissue by excess suction. It is all plastic, lightweight, has two shield sizes and adapts for use with the electric pump. The adaptability of the Medela hand pump is especially valuable for mothers who need the efficiency and convenience of both electric and manual pumping. This pump is available from most breastfeeding centers, lactation consultants, La Leche League, or the Medela Company. The Kaneson/Marshal is also a popular cylindrical-type pump available at most pharmacies, maternity shops, department stores, and stores carrying infant-care items. Good-quality cylindrical pumps sell in the $25 range.

The bulb-type manual pump also called a "bicycle horn" pump, consists of a glass or plastic cup attached to a rubber bulb. These are the least expensive and most widely available type of pump, but we do not recommend them for several reasons: they are usually ineffective in emptying the breast; they are uncomfortable and may damage breast tissue because they have no mechanism for release of the vacuum; the suction strength is very difficult to control; and in some very inexpensive types, the milk can enter the bulb and become contaminated.

Battery-operated breast pumps are a recent advance in improving the effectiveness and comfort of pumping milk. The only advantage of a battery-operated pump is that you don't have to operate it manually. It takes a reasonable amount of manual dexterity to operate a hand pump, and some mothers find this cumbersome. The battery-operated breast pump is helpful for the mother who feels she fumbles a lot with the manually-operated pump. Its only advantage over the electric pump is it can be used when you are away from an electrical outlet. At present the biggest disadvantage of battery pumps is the short life of the batteries and therefore the inconsistent level of suction. A good battery-operated breast pump sells for between $40 and $80, and rechargeable models are becoming increasingly available. Working mothers who pump their milk away from home also find the battery-operated pump to be less cumbersome and time-consuming than the hand pump.

Small electric breast pumps are equivalent to the battery-powered models in cost, size and ease of use and do not need batteries. Their only disadvantage is the need for a wall outlet, which may not always be available.

Large electric breast pumps are the most efficient, comfortable and easiest to use of all pumps. They are designed to simulate a baby's normal sucking pattern as much as possible. The intensity of the suction is also adjustable to your individual level of comfort. Accessories for maximizing the effectiveness and comfort of pumping are more available for large electric pumps than for the other types, and various cup sizes are available. One of the latest innovations is the double pumping mechanism available from Medela; it contains two collecting systems, allowing simultaneous emptying of both breasts. One of the most valuable features of the electric breast pump is that you can do other things while pumping your milk, such as telling a story to an older child, reading a book, or just sitting down and relaxing with one hand free.

Most electric breast pumps were obviously designed by male engineers. They are visually unattractive and do nothing to stimulate maternal instincts. For this reason we recommend pasting a large picture of your baby on or near the pump and that you "think baby" while you are pumping. We strongly recommend the use of electric breast pumps over the other types, as the advantages far outweigh the disadvantages. We usually use electric breast pumps early in the newborn period to get mother's milk established if her baby is not breastfeeding efficiently. Once a good milk flow is established by electric pump, a mother can graduate to the manual pump if cost is a consideration. The disadvantages of the electric pump are its size, weight, and cost. Electric pumps range from car-battery to shoebox size. They are too large and heavy to be carried in a purse, but some of the smaller electric pumps can be carried in a diaper bag. Their purchase price ranges from $400 to $1,000. Most electric breast pumps are rented (averaging $2 a day for short-term rental, down to $1 a day for a five-month term rental). If you plan to pump your milk for a long period of time—say, if you have a premature baby requiring long-term hospitalization or if you are returning to work but wish to continue breastfeeding for quite a while, we recommend using the electric pump together with a manual/electric pump kit.

If you choose an electric breast pump we advise using the double pumping kit available from Medela. Because both breasts are emptied simultaneously, pumping time is cut in half, so working mothers can successfully complete pumping during their regular break (10 to 15 minutes). In addition, research indicates that double pumping significantly increases blood prolactin levels, which help maintain mother's milk supplies. This unexpected side benefit is important to working mothers and mothers of premature infants, who may have difficulty maintaining and increasing milk supply when baby is not available for breast stimulation.

For more information, see the Resources list on page 167.

24

NIGHTTIME BREASTFEEDING

It is the norm rather than the exception for the breastfeeding infant to wake during the night for the first six months and sometimes even the first year. The medical definition of "sleeping through the night" is five straight hours, and babies are not expected to do this until around three months. This is why breastfeeding is called a lifestyle, not just a method of feeding.

Anthropologists have noticed that in cultures that breastfeed nearly exclusively, babies feed almost continuously every few hours around the clock. Babies sleep next to their mothers at night; the nursing pair may breastfeed right through sleep without completely awakening. Experts in infant development believe that the harmony between a mother and her suckling infant has an organizing effect on a baby's sleep pattern. The mother apparently exerts a regulatory effect on the infant's sleep/wake cycle with the periodic delivery of milk. In essence, research is showing that frequent feedings around the clock may be important toward organizing the baby's temperament and in promoting day waking and night sleeping.

Our culture, however, is very oriented toward getting babies to sleep all through the night (8 to 12 hours). In fact, this used to be one of the questions that new parents were often asked by their health care providers—"Is your baby sleeping through the night?"—as if this were a goal to shoot for, and failure to reach it meant that one member of the mother-infant pair was failing to do his or her job. Now that infant-care specialists are beginning to realize that sleeping through the night may indeed not be the "norm," the issue is no longer given such priority. The nature of human milk may give us a clue as to how human infants should be fed and how long a breastfed infant can sleep. Anthropologists who study the feeding patterns of various species have concluded that infants are designed to be fed very frequently, and through the night. Anthropologists have also discovered that the relatively low fat and protein content of human milk requires frequent day and night feedings.

Tiny babies have tiny tummies. This anatomic fact, together with the low fat and protein content of breast milk (making it "less filling"), indicates that breastfeeding babies need night feedings, certainly in the early months.

All science aside, how does a breastfeeding mother get a good night's sleep? In looking through our gallery of successful breastfeeding families we noticed that the great majority of the mothers sleep with their babies at least during the early months. One day during a parenting seminar, I was explaining to a group of breastfeeding mothers all the scientific benefits of sleeping with their babies when one mother exclaimed, "I didn't do it because of all these scientific reasons, I did it for sheer survival!" Consider the following advantages of sleeping with your breastfeeding baby.

Mother and baby sleep better. This is because of the mutual giving effect of "nursing down" (a term we use for breastfeeding off to sleep). We have noticed that our own babies often fade out immediately after a breastfeeding, as if they had been given a shot of sleeping medication. In fact, this may be true; breast milk contains a recently discovered sleep-inducing protein.* Also, the act of breastfeeding stimulates the hormone prolactin to enter the mother's bloodstream and have a tranquilizing effect on her. When the breastfeeding pair drift off to sleep, the mother puts the baby to sleep and the baby puts the mother to sleep. This is especially helpful for mothers who have had a busy schedule during the day and are wound up at night.

Babies grow better. One of the oldest treatments for the slow-gaining baby is night nursing. Some mothers tell us that they experience a stronger milk ejection reflex at night; perhaps this is due to the fact that they are more relaxed. A more efficient milk ejection reflex would give night nursers milk higher in fat and thus higher in the calories that they need to grow. Some researchers believe that the closeness to the mother, the skin-to-skin contact, may stimulate the mother to produce more growth hormone; this has been found to be true in experimental animals.

Mothers' prolactin levels are higher during sleep. Since prolactin is the primary hormone involved in milk production, the quantity of breast milk available should be greater when baby sucks at night. In cultures practicing unrestricted breastfeeding, studies have shown that infants obtain as many of their daily calories during the night as they do during the day. Growth hormone is also secreted mostly at night in babies and children. If babies are meant to grow at night, aren't they also meant to eat at night?

Sharing sleep and nighttime breastfeeding may decrease night waking. When infants and mothers share sleep they achieve nighttime harmony. Picture how this happens: because of the predominance of light sleep cycles, all infants

*Graf, M.V., et al., Presence of Delta Sleep-inducing Peptide-like Material in Human Milk. *J Clin Endocrinol Metab* 59:127, 1984.

are prone to frequent night waking during the first six months. As the infant ascends from the state of deep sleep into the state of light sleep, he passes through a vulnerable period in which he often awakens. When babies and mothers share sleep, they get their sleep cycles in harmony with each other. Babies and mothers share deep and light sleep cycles so that, when baby ascends from the state of deep sleep into the state of light sleep and enters into the vulnerable period for night waking, mother also partially awakens and nurses her baby through this vulnerable period. It is not how often one is awakened that makes for a "wiped out feeling" the next day; it is how one is awakened. Picture what happens if mother and baby sleep separately, for example, in separate rooms. The hungry baby wakes up and cries for mother. Because mother is not immediately next to him, he has to cry louder in order to get mother's attention. By the time mother arrives to offer the breast to comfort the crying baby, she is groggy, wakened from a deep sleep, and often angry; baby is anxious and it takes longer for baby and mother to resettle into sleep. Why? Because their sleep cycles are out of sync. Admittedly, this nighttime harmony does not always work and some babies and mothers do sleep better separately. But when it does work, it works beautifully; it is certainly worth a try to achieve it.

Other ways of helping baby and mother get a good night's sleep. Around the third or fourth month a baby sometimes gets into the exhausting habit of becoming a day player and night nurser. Babies at this age are so attracted by the ability to see across the room and relate to interesting visual stimuli that they "forget" to nurse during the day. We call them "Mr. Suck a Little, Look a Little." At night, however, baby's environment is quiet and less interesting, so he settles down to "tank up" on feedings he should have had during the day. To lessen this exhausting habit, purposely "tank up" your baby during the day. Nurse in a dark and uninteresting room, a trick called **sheltered nursing.** In our family of seven we have had to do this because of all the other siblings clamoring for attention and disturbing the little nurser. Otherwise mother may become an all-night diner who is trying to be a good nighttime mother—but she is so tired during the day that she cannot be a good *daytime* mother. Usually the whole family loses when this happens.

Another reason for frequent night waking is the growth spurts that babies undergo, usually around three weeks, six weeks and three months. Because they need more milk during these growth spurts, they marathon nurse day and night for a few days until the increased sucking has produced a higher milk supply.

Studies have shown that breastfed babies do, in fact, wake up more often then formula-fed babies. I suspect there are two reasons for this: the type of milk, breast milk being less filling than formula, and the mother's responsiveness. Because of the increased sensitivity of breastfeeding mothers, they are usually unable to let their babies cry at night and will allow unrestricted nighttime nursing. In an editorial comment about this study, Dr. Dana Raphael, director of the Human Lactation Center in Westport, Connecticut, commented: "There is implicit in the discussion of night waking the idea that something sacred and healthful will occur if a mother and the infant sleep eight straight hours. . . . I would suggest that the problem is in the expectations and anxieties of our culture about sleep. . . . I reckon the problem to be centered right in the middle of an alarm clock. It certainly reflects the social systems so arranged that women have to be up to serve breakfast, run all the household errands, clean, wash, cook, baby tend, etc. without the support of others. These are the culprit facts which make night feeding a problem. The infant and mother have very little to do with it."

What about the frequent night feeder who is beautifully thriving while mother is barely surviving? Picture the following very common scenario: Because baby is such a frequent night nurser, mother and baby sleep together, often for sheer survival, and this arrangement works for the first few months. Mother feels she can tolerate anything in the beginning because sooner or later baby will sleep through the night. Now baby is six months old and still night nursing. Nine months and still night nursing. Mother is getting increasingly exhausted and admits that she is no longer enjoying this style of mothering—"But my baby needs me at night and I can't let her cry." Mother is giving, giving, giving until she gives out and the whole family suffers.

This situation actually occurred in our family during the writing of this book. Here is how we solved it. I first had to convince Martha that she was giving out (while I have great respect for mother's intuition, there is one Achilles heel—they don't recognize when they are giving out). I slept with Stephen for three nights, and when he awakened I rocked him or carried him in a sling until he fell back to sleep again. This did not always work, but it worked most of the time. After three nights he did not awaken to breastfeed as often. Family nighttime harmony was restored. Whether or not night nursing is a need or a habit no one knows, sometimes not even the mother; but even in the most loving households and among the best of parents, some conditioning to sleep is necessary for nighttime breastfeeders. Without this conditioning, some babies will suck through the night for years. There must be a balance in all parenting styles, especially at night.

25

HELPING A BREASTFEEDING BABY TAKE A BOTTLE

While some breastfeeding babies will readily accept an occasional bottle, some little breastfeeding purists will accept no substitute for the real thing. If your family situation warrants the use of an occasional bottle, here is how to make it easier on yourself and your baby.

Beware of the advice to start giving your baby a bottle once a day right after birth "so he will get used to it." Admittedly a bottle a day may not bother some babies, but others will get nipple-confused during the first few weeks. Even one bottle a day can be enough to throw off the supply-and-demand harmony that is so important as babies and mothers are getting the right start. Wait to give the bottles until you need to.

Since it is common for a baby to refuse a bottle from the mother—this is foreign to a baby's feeding program—have someone else introduce it. Initially this should be someone experienced in bottle-feeding babies, such as a grandmother, infant-care nurse or another mother. Such a person has confidence in offering a bottle to a baby, and babies often sense the experience and confidence of the bottle feeder. It is normal for a breastfeeding mother to feel a bit awkward in offering her baby a bottle, and the baby may sense the mother's ambivalence. After baby has learned to accept the bottle from an experienced bottle feeder, father is next in line as the ideal bottle feeder.

The baby should be held and interacted with just as he is during breastfeeding. The caregiver can undress baby for skin-to-skin contact and should maintain eye contact during feeding. The person feeding the baby should convey enjoyment of the interaction. Remember, feeding is not only giving milk but enjoying social interaction. There should always be a person at both ends of the bottle. Avoid bottle propping; leaving the baby unattended in a crib to take his own bottle is actually unsafe. If baby is reluctant to take the bottle, gently stimulate his mouth with the nipple as during breastfeeding. Let the baby "mouth" the bottle nipple to become familiar with it. You may need to experiment with different types of nipples, some being softer and longer than others. The orthodontic-style nipple may be the least confusing. Try varying the nipple temperature; some babies like rubber nipples warm (run warm water over them), while others, such as teething babies, like a cold nipple refrigerator-cold. Also experiment with different hole sizes. Ideally, milk should drip about one drop per second from a full, unshaken bottle held upside down.

Some babies take a bottle better in the usual breastfeeding position; others prefer it in a totally different position because the breastfeeding position may confuse them. They expect the breast and are given a bottle, which may result in an angry protest.

What is in the bottle is as important to a baby as how he gets it. You have four choices: breast milk, formula, diluted apple juice, or water. The ideal is pumped breast milk, as this substance is most familiar to baby, is best in nourishment, and has the sweetest, most pleasant taste. If you are unable to give your baby pumped breast milk in a bottle, try various formulas. Remember always to mix the formula according to directions. It is all right to occasionally dilute the formula, but never make it more concentrated than the directions suggest.

Some breastfeeding babies will not take a bottle while held by a seated person. This reminds them too much of the whole atmosphere of breastfeeding and they will not accept an alternative. Put such a baby in a sling-type carrier and walk around with him while offering a bottle. Try different rocking and moving motions to calm baby before enticing him to take the bottle.

If a baby refuses the bottle despite trying all of the above, relax! He can be fed milk in other ways. If the baby is still young enough to accept a finger into his mouth and suck well, he can be finger fed using a large syringe. If that process is too painstaking or awkward for the caregiver (it's actually easy once you get the hang of it), there are more options. Even a very young baby can be fed milk from a shallow, flexible bowl or from a small-diameter cup, such as a small juice cup or even a medicine cup. This is a bit messy compared to using a bottle, but that's what bibs are for. Hold the baby up at a good angle, supporting his head and neck with your hand, and carefully tip the bowl or cup up to his lips. He'll get a taste and eagerly lick at the milk. Patiently allow him to learn to lap the milk and swallow it. There is a trainer cup on the market, made by Infa, that is a bottle with a drinking rim on top instead of a nipple. This may be a good tool to use if you have a baby who will only sip his milk.

26

BREASTFEEDING AND WORKING

Some mothers automatically consider breastfeeding and working incompatible. Breastfeeding, however, may be even more important for the working mother for the following reasons. Breastfeeding alleviates some of the guilt stemming from leaving your baby, since he gets your milk, although from a bottle, when you are not there. Breastfeeding provides a unique mother-infant attachment that a babysitter cannot give your child, and adds an element of consistency to caregiving. Breastfeeding and working is one of the many "juggling" acts that enable a mother to adapt to changing times, yet meet some of her own basic needs and follow her intuition. Here is how to enjoy breastfeeding and working.

Plan ahead. While it is necessary to plan ahead, do not overfocus on "the day I have to go back to work." Working mothers have confided in me that this subconsciously dilutes their attachment to their baby in order to make it easier for them to leave. Try to extend your maternity leave as long as possible. Both you and your baby deserve this.

Choose substitute baby care wisely. Get your babysitter familiar with your baby starting around two weeks before you go back to work, so they are not strangers. Arrange for several visits for the three of you, and use that time to gradually let her know what you want from her. Choose a caregiver who has the same attachment values that you do. Ask her, "What will you do when my baby cries?" Choose someone who will give a nurturant response to your crying baby.

Discuss your breastfeeding arrangement with your employer. If he or she objects to this intrusion into your work, obtain a doctor's note that you should breastfeed your baby. If you can, have an arrangement whereby baby can be brought to you for breastfeeding at your work or at least that you have time off to pump and store your milk. In recent test cases in the United States, the courts have upheld the mothers' right to breastfeed babies while on the job. Employers, courts and unions do not like the image that they are against mothering. Society is finally recognizing that human milk for human babies is a valuable natural resource. Everyone will be on your side. Give your employer two messages: breastfeeding is important to you; a content employee is a productive employee. Also let him know that you will not allow breastfeeding to interfere with your work. Consider this dilemma from your employer's viewpoint: he has the responsibility to be sure a certain amount of work is done by each employee. It is up to you to convince your employer that breastfeeding will not detract from your performance.

At this writing, a woman named Kathy, one of our office staff, brings her baby to work. She had to return to work for economic reasons but felt intuitively that she simply could not leave and wean her baby. I sensed her need to work and her need to mother. She sensed my need for a certain amount of work to be done. We devised a solution where all three of our needs are met—hers, mine, and baby's. There are days when her baby is particularly fussy and her work is compromised. She makes up for this added time with her baby by giving added time to her job.

Work and wear. Besides the option of leaving your baby

with a substitute caregiver and breastfeeding part-time, consider one of the latest innovations in the marketplace—work and wear. If you have the kind of job that allows you to take your baby with you, get a sling-type carrier (I recommend Nojo's baby sling) and "wear" your baby to work. Many mothers in our practice do this. They have jobs as house cleaners, real estate agents, salesclerks in baby and department stores, and even kindergarten teachers. Work and wear is how mothers the world over have always incorporated their mothering and working. Finally this beautiful custom has arrived in the Western world. When I watch Kathy wear her baby Elizabeth in our office, I am impressed by how much Elizabeth learns by "working with mother." Every word that Kathy says, Elizabeth hears. Every task that mother performs, baby sees. Baby is intimately involved in the world of the mother, later to be the world of the baby. Besides promoting mother-infant attachment, working and wearing humanizes the baby.

Introducing the bottle. It's true—the longer you wait to introduce the bottle, the less she will want to take it. With some babies, if you introduce the bottle too early (in the first week) they will develop nipple confusion and breastfeed poorly. We usually recommend introducing the bottle two weeks before going back to work, or at least by six weeks of age. Have someone else offer the baby the bottle, as it is very common for baby to refuse to accept a bottle from mother.

Storing up a milk supply. It is wise to begin pumping and storing a supply of your breast milk before returning to work. Some babies either refuse to take formula or are allergic to all the commercial formulas and will only thrive on your breast milk. If you have pumped and stored a supply of your milk before returning to work, this problem will be alleviated. Stockpiling a supply of your milk in the freezer is a valuable investment into the future nutrition and health of your baby.

What to expect. When you begin pumping your milk, don't be discouraged if you obtain only a small amount at first. With practice, most mothers are able to pump several ounces within 10 or 15 minutes. It is normal for the amount to vary from one pumping session to the next and to experience high-production and low-production days. In the first week after returning to work, expect your breasts to leak milk at inconvenient times. Discreetly fold your arms across your breasts and apply pressure directly to your nipples for a minute or two. Wear breast pads and change them often. As your milk production system is getting adjusted to a new timer, expect periodic engorgement at "feeding times" during the first week or two. This nuisance and discomfort will subside as you develop a pumping routine while away from your baby.

Tools you will need. To make breastfeeding and working easier, you will need the following equipment:

- A breast pump,either manual or electric.
- Breast pads.
- A tote bag for your pump (if you don't leave it at work) and the milk containers and cooler.

Wardrobe tips for the working breastfeeding mother. Wear print blouses or tops that will not show any leaking and won't show the outline of your nipples or breast pads. Whites, dark solids and pale colors may show leaking. Wear breast pads in your bra for the first few weeks and change them whenever they get wet. Cotton and synthetic fabrics do not show leaking as much as silks, which are easily stained. Loose breastfeeding blouses will be much more attractive then clinging materials (see Key 15 for more wardrobe tips).

Collecting milk while at work. At least every three hours, pump as much milk as you can and store it in the refrigerator. If you are unable to take time off during your regular schedule to pump your milk, collect your milk during coffee breaks or lunch breaks. Look at a picture of your baby while pumping your milk, as this gets your milk-producing hormones running and activates the milk ejection reflex, making pumping more productive. Use of a double pumping system will cut pumping time in half (see Key 23).

Your schedule during breastfeeding while working. Have a happy departure and a happy reunion. Breastfeed your baby before leaving for work and as soon as you return home. Leave instructions for the sitter not to feed the baby within an hour before you return home so that your baby is eager to feed and have a happy reunion. After you return to work, expect your baby to become a night nurser. A very common breastfeeding pattern when mothers return to work is for baby to feed less frequently during the day from the substitute caregiver and more frequently at night from mother. Experienced mothers who have successfully managed breastfeeding while working have found it easier to accept this as a natural part of working and mothering; they simply take their baby to bed and enjoy night nursing. The extra touch time and interaction helps compensate for the time apart. On weekends, holidays, and days off, return to full-time breastfeeding; periodic full nursing days are necessary to keep milk production adequate. If you have been full-time breastfeeding over the weekend, expect your breasts to be fuller than usual on Monday. The ultimate in nighttime harmony is to be able to breastfeed your baby at night without either member of the nursing pair completely awakening. The relaxing effects of night nursing also help mothers unwind from a busy day.

Try to make it as easy as possible for your caregiver to feed your baby. Try the following tips:

1. Be sure your sitter holds your baby in the breastfeeding position while giving a bottle. Do not allow

her to prop the bottle and leave baby unattended. (If this is her style, she's not nurturing enough for your baby.)

2. Refrigerated breast milk is not homogenized and will separate. Instruct the sitter to shake gently to mix the milk while warming it in a bowl of very warm water.
3. If baby seems hungry just before mother is due home, try to keep him distracted with play or satisfied with just a small amount of milk so he is not filled up when mother arrives.
4. Instruct your caregiver how to heat stored breast milk. Do not heat the milk in a microwave, as it will destroy valuable nutrients. Thaw only a few ounces at a time. To thaw frozen milk, hold the container under cool running water and gradually add warmer water until the milk is thawed and heated to room temperature. Thawed milk cannot be refrozen, so freeze it in small—2- or 4-ounce—amounts.

What's in it for you? We highly encourage our own patients to continue breastfeeding when returning to work. At The Breastfeeding Center we even have had several airline stewardesses who are away from their babies for two or three days at a time but have managed to continue a part-time breastfeeding relationship for two years. Mothers who breastfeed and work report an enhanced closeness and sensitivity toward their baby. They also notice the relaxing effects of breastfeeding. One mother stated, "I have a very stressful job, and I'm very tense when I return home. I settle down and breastfeed my baby. She feels better and I feel better. What a happy reunion!"

27

STORING AND TRANSPORTING BREAST MILK

It is wise to stockpile some of your breastmilk in case you experience an illness and are unable to breastfeed, are returning to work, or will be away from your baby and need your milk to be given by a substitute caregiver. The following information is correct if your baby is healthy and full-term. Milk collected and stored for a hospitalized baby will need further guidelines, so check with the nurses. You must wash your hands before collecting your milk and wash containers in hot, soapy water and rinse well.

Containers. There are two types of containers for storing milk, plastic and glass. Research suggests that plastic is better than glass for two reasons: glass breaks, and some of the white blood cells in breast milk cling to the glass, but cling less to plastic. The disposable 4-ounce nurser bags used for bottle feeding are very convenient to store breast milk. It is best to store the milk in 4-ounce containers rather than larger ones; this makes thawing easier and wastes less milk.

Once breast milk is thawed it should not be refrozen. Label each container with the date; when using disposable plastic nursers, use double bags in case the outside bag tears. Some breastfeeding centers recommend using heavy plastic containers to store milk for long periods of time, since the plastic bags may split when frozen and then absorb odors from nearby foods. Leave an inch of space in the bag or bottle on top of the milk, as milk expands as it freezes. It is wise to have a few containers filled with only 2 ounces of milk in case a babysitter needs some until mother returns.

How long milk keeps. Expressed breast milk may be given to baby within 30 minutes without any special storage. Breast milk may be safely kept unrefrigerated in a **sterilized container** for up to six hours, if you are traveling and refrigeration is impossible. But unless refrigeration is impossible, do not leave breast milk unrefrigerated for more than 30 minutes. Breast milk may be stored in a refrigerator for up to five days before use; after that it should be frozen. Milk can be kept in the freezer section of a refrigerator for two weeks, or in a freezer with a separate door for up to four months. For long-term storage—six months or more—a deep freeze at a constant 0°F is best. Be sure to date the milk and use up the older milk first. Breastfeeding centers do not recommend keeping frozen breast milk for longer than six months.

You can add expressed breast milk to milk that is already frozen. *Be sure to chill the milk first in the refrigerator;* adding warm milk can defrost the top layer of the frozen milk. If you have more than 2 ounces to add, it is best to use a separate container.

Cleaning and sterilizing. A dishwasher that uses a water temperature of at least 180°F will sterilize everything well enough. If you do not use a dishwasher, try the following: Pad the bottom of a large pot with a dishcloth or towel and place bottles, nipples, cups, etc., on the pad. Fill the pot with enough water to completely cover the items you are sterilizing. Bring the water to a boil over high heat and then turn down the heat just enough so the water continues to boil gently. Boil for 5 minutes. Remove the rubber nipples with sterile tongs and place them on a clean towel. Allow all the other items to boil for 15 minutes longer. Do not touch the rims of the bottles or the insides of the caps with your hands.

Defrosting milk. Do not thaw frozen milk on top of the stove; it will curdle. Do not heat either breast milk or formula in a microwave oven because the uneven heat may cause hot spots, and valuable nutrients are destroyed. In fact, researchers at the University of Vienna found that microwaving protein foods such as cheese, meat, and fish changes several amino acids to molecular "toxic mirror images" that can actually destroy nerve cells (this study was published in *Lancet*, December 9, 1989). Also avoid heating milk in a pan of warm water on a stove since it is easy to forget the milk is there, leading to overheating, boiling over, and wasted milk. The best and safest way to thaw or heat expressed milk is under running water. Place the bag or bottle of milk upright in a bowl and run water over it, gradually increasing the temperature until it becomes warm. As you warm the milk, gently shake the bag to mix the separated cream and milk. Shake the bottle of milk again before feeding. If your baby does not take all of the thawed milk, you can use defrosted and refrigerated milk within 12 hours; don't refreeze it. Put only a few ounces of the milk in the bottle at any one time, then add to it if necessary. It is unwise to offer baby the rest of the bottle of unused breast milk since his saliva may have mixed with the milk and contaminated it.

Transporting expressed milk. A thermos bottle or an insulated bag filled with ice packs is best for transporting milk. Special insulated bags for this purpose are available from La Leche. If you have pumped your milk at the office, refrigerate it first before putting it in a thermos, or put it in a container in your special bag and surround it with cold packs. Mothers who transport it from work to home take great care to protect their cargo.

28

FATHER'S ROLE

Many fathers feel left out of the inner circle of breastfeeding. The father does, in fact, play an extremely important part in it. When reviewing our patients to determine what contributes to successful breastfeeding, one factor stands out—a sensitive and supportive father.

Martha decided to breastfeed our first child back in the 1960s, when only about 25% of women chose to breastfeed. I was a pediatric intern at that time and didn't know much about the advantages of breast milk. I didn't offer an opinion for or against the idea and provided, at best, only passive encouragement. Now, after 25 years of marriage, seven breastfed children and 20 years in pediatric practice, I am absolutely convinced of its value. For this reason I want to convey to new fathers a very important message: *Do everything within your power to encourage and support breastfeeding. Providing understanding and support for the breastfeeding pair is one of the most valuable investments you can make in their health and well-being.*

The care and feeding of the mother. Dads, remember that a breastfeeding mother is biologically programmed to give, give, give. This is especially true if you are blessed with a high-need baby. With this type of baby, mother keeps giving, baby keeps taking. Baby thrives but mom barely survives. The problem is that mothers keep giving and do not realize they are giving out. Mothers who are most on fire are the ones who most easily burn out. Father's main roles in the breastfeeding relationship are: to support the breastfeeding mother, relieving her of the many household tasks that drain her energy; and to develop comforting skills to calm your baby during those high-need periods.

Develop comforting skills. The following scenario is very common among breastfeeding mothers and their infants. Every time baby cries, mother picks him up and nurses him. This interaction may be repeated five to ten times a day. It usually works; an upset baby will nearly always calm down when put to the breast. Because this calming technique works so well, father leaves all the comforting skills to mother. Also, because mother becomes such an effective comforter and father never learns comforting skills, mother is afraid to leave baby in the care of her husband. Even when she does, she hovers around and as soon as baby starts to cry she "rescues" him from the father—who by this time feels well-meaning but bumbling. In this typical scenario (it used to happen in our family too), all family members lose a bit. Dad never gets a chance to develop comforting skills, baby never gets used to dad's unique method of comforting, and mother never gets a break.

Try the following holding patterns as soon as possible:

The neck nestle. Nestle your baby's head against the front of your neck and drape your throat area right over baby's skull. Sing a droning song like *Old Man River.* The male voice vibrates more than the female, and a tiny baby hears with the vibration of her skull bones and eardrums. By using the neck nestle and singing to her, you will find a very effective way of comforting her.

The warm fuzzy is another male comforting measure. Drape baby, skin to skin, over your chest with her ear over your heartbeat. The rise and fall of your chest during your breathing motions will usually lull baby right to sleep.

Wear your baby. Put your baby in a sling-type carrier and wear her as much as possible so that baby gets used to the rhythm of your walk, your sound, and your dance.

Freeway fathering is another way of comforting the upset baby. Place your baby in a car seat and take a long nonstop drive, meanwhile insisting your wife do something for herself. Babies usually fall asleep during long rides.

Try these above comforting measures very early. Mothers have a natural protective instinct about their babies, feeling that no one else can comfort them as well as they can. The "my baby needs me" attitude is normal. The father has to prove himself as a baby comforter in order for mother to feel comfortable to release "her baby" to the care of dad.

Be sensitive. Realize that a breastfeeding mother may experience many mood swings because of the hormonal changes and because of extreme fatigue. One mother confided in me, "I'd have to hit my husband over the head before he realized I'm giving out." Ask your wife what she needs and how you can help. Don't expect her to volunteer that she needs help, because this may weaken the supermom myth. Take inventory of everything that saps your wife's energy and diverts it from breastfeeding. Take over as many of these tasks as you can, delegate them to the other children, or hire help.

Encourage your wife to do something just for herself—something relaxing that she enjoys. Make an appointment for her and drive her there, letting her know that you really care about her relaxing. Remember that you have to purposely overcome the "my baby needs me so much, I can't leave her" feeling that most breastfeeding mothers have. As one father of a breastfeeding family summed it up very wisely, "I can't breastfeed our baby, but I can create an environment that helps my wife breastfeed better."

29

INTRODUCING SOLID FOODS

If your infant is thriving and neither you nor baby has any interest in solids, then don't be in a hurry to introduce them. While most babies do enjoy some solid foods by six months of age, some babies, especially breastfed ones, are content with only breast milk and don't need or want solids for a few more months. In our experience, breastfeeding mothers often start solids later than do bottle-feeding mothers. Probably the reason for this difference is that bottle-feeding mothers, because they can count ounces, seem more time-oriented during infant feeding. If their baby seems to take more formula more frequently, mothers often interpret this as a sign of needing solid foods, whereas breastfeeding mothers simply nurse more to accommodate baby.

It is wise to feed your baby according to his own developmental stage of feeding readiness, not according to some predetermined age. Here's how to notice when your baby is ready for solid foods.

Watch for signs of interest: baby may watch you eat, following your fork from your plate to your mouth. Watch for "begging" signs: baby will reach out and grab some of your food. Watch for signs of developmental readiness: baby is able to sit up in a high chair and pick up food with his hands. An important developmental milestone of feeding readiness is the diminishing of the tongue-thrusting reflex. When a foreign substance is placed upon an infant's tongue, it reflexively pushes the substance out, protecting baby against choking. This reflex diminishes around six months, enabling baby to handle solid foods. Another sign of readiness is that baby seems not to be satisfied with only your milk. After two or three days of increased breastfeeding he is not satisfied, he wants to feed more frequently, wakes up more often, and shows signs of interest in something more than your milk.

If your baby is content to receive his nutrition all prepackaged and delivered in a way that he enjoys, then don't force solids. The reason we wait for baby to show interest in solids is to capitalize on a basic principle of learning: any developmental skill is best learned when it is initiated by the baby. When your baby initiates signs of readiness, it's time to begin.

When you notice signs of readiness for solid food, start with solids that are closest to your milk in taste and consistency. A very ripe banana—sweet and smooth like your milk—is a good starter food. Remember, your baby has to develop an entirely new feeding mechanism, from suck-swallow to tongue-mashing and swallowing. Start with a fingertip of mashed banana as a test dose. Place a small dollop of banana on the tip of your baby's tongue, allowing him to get used to handling the new texture and taste. If you put the first solid food too far back, this may confuse your baby and cause difficulty in swallowing. If the banana goes in, your baby is ready; if the banana comes back at you, baby is not interested. Start with about a teaspoon of each new food. Remember that your initial goal is to introduce your baby to new tastes, new textures, not to fill him up. Gradually vary the texture and amount to fit the eating skills and appetite of your baby. Some like solids of thinner consistency and want a larger amount. Some do better with thicker solids and smaller amounts.

Observe "stop signs" as well: pursed lips, closed mouth, head turning away when the spoon is coming toward him are all signals that baby does not want to eat right now. Don't force feed. You want your baby to develop a healthy attitude both toward the food and the feeding, and it helps if you develop a healthy attitude about infant feeding yourself. When beginning solids, think of feeding as helping your baby to develop a new skill that you want him to enjoy. Don't be preoccupied with how much your baby takes. Offer solids at the time of the day when the baby seems hungriest and most bored, and when your milk is the lowest—usually toward the end of the day. Since infants have no concept of breakfast, lunch, or dinner, it really makes no difference when they receive what. Bananas, rice or barley cereal, applesauce, peaches, pears, carrots, squash, sweet potatoes, mashed potatoes and avocados are all favorite starter foods.

Besides using your fingertip or a spoon to start solids, allow your baby to feed himself. Place a bit of mashed banana within grabbing distance on his table or high-chair tray; this will also help make the most of his rapidly developing hand skills. At around six months, babies pounce upon anything of interest placed in front of them. You will notice that your baby will soon pick up a morsel of food between thumb and fingers and gradually zero in on his mouth. At first the baby may show more misses than hits, resulting in the food splattering all over his cheeks—but sharing the food with face and bib is part of the feeding game. Allow your baby to experience some trial and error; eventually practice makes perfect.

Many breastfeeding mothers delay solids as long as possible because of a family history of allergy. This is wise because the older the baby, the more mature his intestines and the more likely that they will be able to filter out allergenic proteins or digest them into smaller, less allergenic molecules. The starter foods least likely to cause allergies are bananas, rice or barley cereal, carrots, squash, sweet potatoes, avocado, and mashed potatoes (made without cow's milk). Avoid mixed cereals and, for that matter, any packaged mixtures, because if your baby is allergic, it is more difficult to identify the allergen in mixed foods. Avoid egg yolk before nine months and egg white before one year. Delay dairy products as long as possible. It is wise to space each new food about a week apart and to keep a diary of which foods your baby may be allergic to; if baby is allergic to any foods in your diet (through your breast milk), you have a clue that he may be allergic to the same solid foods (see Key 18 for diet during breastfeeding). The usual signs of food allergies are bloating and gassiness, a sandpaperlike rash on the face, a runny nose and watery eyes, diarrhea and diaper rash, night waking and general cranky behavior. Sometimes around four or five months babies go through a growth spurt and they want to marathon nurse every few hours around the clock for one or two days. Mothers sometimes interpret this as a sign of solid-food readiness. It may well be, but sometimes baby does not need solids—just a couple of days of increased nursing and he will settle down to his previous routine.

Because breastfed babies enjoy night nursing, mothers may be tempted to try filling a baby up with solid food before bedtime in hopes that he will sleep through the night. Controlled studies with same-aged babies in which one group was given solid foods before bedtime and the other group was only formula- or breastfed, found that there was no difference in the amount of night waking. As parents of seven, we too, have periodically tried "filler feeding" but have found it ineffective.

Reading your baby's breastfeeding cues, encouraging self feeding, and advancing gradually all lead to creating a healthy feeding attitude. To a baby, eating is not only a nutritional necessity but a developmental skill. The more a baby enjoys practicing a skill the more efficiently he will advance in it. Infant feeding not only provides fun and nutrition for a baby but also helps parents witness and enjoy their baby's rapidly developing manual skills. Feeding is a social interaction, not just a nutritional necessity. Enjoy it!

Remember that beverages, such as juice, should be an *addition* to breastfeeding, not a substitute for it. Consider your breast milk as a food and a beverage, and don't be in a hurry to introduce juice.

30

COMMON NURSING CHALLENGES

Nursing strike. Your baby may temporarily lose interest in nursing for a few days, but please don't immediately interpret this as time for weaning. For a variety of reasons, some babies periodically refuse to breastfeed for a day or two, and then resume their previous breastfeeding routine. This is humorously called a "nursing strike," and it has the following causes:

Physical upsets such as a cold, teething, change in routine, hospitalization, or fever may cause a baby to either have a greater desire for breastfeeding or to go on a nursing strike. Our first baby, Jim, refused to breastfeed after a trip to the emergency room for stitches following a fall at eight months of age. Being young parents, we interpreted this as his time to wean—after all, he was eight months old and in those days nearly all babies were weaned by eight months. He also ate three meals of solids by then and drank well from a cup, so we made no attempts to encourage him back to the breast. We now know that this was a nursing strike.

Emotional upsets such as a recent move, illness in the mother, or family discord may result in a nursing strike. Sometimes the "busy nest syndrome" (too many visitors, too many outside responsibilities, too much holiday stress, etc.) may result in baby temporarily losing interest in nursing.

Overcoming the nursing strike. First, recognize that this is a temporary loss of interest and not a sign that your baby is ready to wean permanently. Rarely does a baby under nine months of age want to wean from the breast. As a general guide, if baby loses interest in nursing and is less than nine months old, first consider it a nursing strike. Older babies go on nursing strikes, too, and only time and effort will tell if he'll nurse again.

The key to overcoming a nursing strike is to woo baby back to the breast. Have a family council with your husband and the rest of the children and explain the situation to them. Temporarily shelve as many outside responsibilities as you can. Delegate the housework, the cooking, and any other chores that can be done by someone else. "Pretend" that you are just beginning to breastfeed your baby and start all over again. Take the telephone off the hook. Sit down at a comfortable nursing station (see Key 16 for how to prepare a nursing station). Turn on some soothing music and sit there and nurse, or just hold your baby most of the day. Soak in the tub together. Wear your baby in a sling-type carrier as much as possible during the day to keep him close to your breast. Nap nursing and night nursing are surefire ways to woo baby back to the breast; periodically during the day lie down on your bed, snuggle up next to your baby and nurse. Take the baby to bed with you at night and allow some nighttime closeness. Babies who resist nursing when awake will often nurse well when drowsy or even asleep! Sometimes just recreating the whole atmosphere of nursing reminds baby of the ambiance of the breastfeeding relationship, and he will feel his resistance weaken.

If baby withdraws from your breast, don't force the feeding. Let baby fall asleep, skin to skin with his head nestling on your breast. Try to duplicate the nursing environment you and your baby enjoyed before the strike. A nursing strike may be baby's message that he wants to renegotiate the mother-infant contract. With a little perseverance and increased attachment, most of these strikes are over within a few days. We have known babies who refused for nearly a week, then only gradually came back to a comfortable nursing situation. These mothers hung in there, made themselves ultra-available, pumped to maintain a milk supply and followed their intuition that their baby was really not ready to wean. If, after all that, baby does wean, it is reassuring to know that it truly was baby's idea and he is, in fact, ready to move on to a new level of maturity. There should be no regret here—just know that your baby was "ripe" ahead of schedule. The two of you will plunge into the next phase of life with just as much gusto as you enjoyed the one that has passed.

The distracted nurser. Sometime between three and six months of age, expect your baby to nurse for a few minutes, pull away, nurse for another few minutes, and pull away again. This common nursing nuisance is mainly due to the rapid development of your baby's visual acuity. By this age he is able to see things very clearly across the room and he notices passersby. He is so distracted by all the goings-on in his increasingly interesting environment that he pauses frequently to attend to something visually appealing. We call this nuisance, "Mr.-Suck-A-Little, Look-A-Little." Experienced breastfeeding mothers have handled this nursing nuisance by "sheltered nursing." Several times a day take your baby into a dark, quiet, and uninteresting room and get down to the business of nursing. Nap nurse more frequently, since at nap-time baby is usually more interested in his immediate environment—namely mother. Swaddling your baby will keep his limbs from swinging during nursing. Wearing the baby in a sling-type carrier and pulling the sling up over him during nursing will keep the distracted nurser from flinging his head back to explore his environment—and taking your breast with him. This is a passing nuisance which the above creative feeding techniques and a bit of humor will solve. He'll soon discover that he can nurse and look at the same time.

Marathoning. In the first few months babies have "frequency days" when all they want to do is nurse—appropriately called marathon nursing. The supply-and-demand principle of breastfeeding is working in response to a growth spurt, most common around three weeks, six weeks, three months, and six months. The baby nurses more in order to stimulate you to produce more so he can grow faster. Your baby may also be going through a period of high need. Some so-called "high-need babies" want to be held "all the time" and nursed "all the time" during the first few months, as they are slowly becoming adjusted to life outside the womb.

During high-need days, temporarily shelve all the outside commitments that may drain your energy. Your baby is only a baby for a very short while, and no one's life is going to be affected if the housework doesn't get done on time. In our experience, mothers become burned out from marathon nursing not so much because of the demands of their baby, but because of too many other family commitments.

Be sure your baby is getting mostly milk at each feeding, not a lot of air. He should be latching on to your areola and should have a good seal. Burp him well during and after a feeding. Use the burp-and-switch technique to attempt to get more of the higher-fat milk into your baby to satisfy him longer. Get used to "wearing" your baby in a sling. This not only makes nursing more accessible, but it may be that your high-need baby wants the comfort of your closeness even more than the milk. Avoid the "filler food" fallacy. You may be advised to give your baby a supplemental bottle or cereal with the implication that you don't have enough milk, but this is usually not necessary. Your baby is simply signaling that he needs to nurse more, and you need to increase your level of supply to meet his level of need. Sleep when your baby sleeps and don't be tempted to "finally get something done." You need to recharge your own system to cope with these high-need periods. Like all the other nursing challenges, this marathon nursing pattern will soon pass.

The biter. I (Martha) have survived 15 years of nursing our seven occasional biters. The usual reaction is to pull baby away from the breast and scream "no." But some mothers are so violent in their reaction to being bitten (and you can hardly blame them if it's a good hard bite) that baby is frightened and may refuse to finish feeding. Instead of pulling your baby away, try this: Pull your baby in very close to you when you sense that his teeth are coming down and you feel the bite. Draw him right into your breast. He will automatically let go in order to open his mouth more to breathe. If he still bites, put your finger between his teeth and your nipple and gently ease him off the breast. Sooner or later baby will realize that each time he bites he gets an undesirable reaction. It is okay to say no, but try your best not to screech in agony because you really can startle your baby enough to put him off nursing for a few days. Keep a record of when he usually bites. If he is doing it at the end of the feeding, interrupt the feeding before he has a chance to clamp down. Also keep some chilled teething toys, a cold washcloth, or a frozen banana on hand and let him chomp on these toward the end of the feeding. Or let him teethe on an inanimate object *before* the feeding, if he bites right at the beginning of nursing. These techniques plus saying, "Ouch, that hurts mama!" will help preserve your breast and teach your baby at the same time.

31

MEDICATIONS WHILE BREASTFEEDING

The information provided in this Key is meant only as a guide. New information concerning the potential safety or harm of a drug may emerge after this writing. For this reason it is advisable to check with your doctor before taking any drug while breastfeeding.

At some time during breastfeeding you may need to take medications. Almost every drug taken by the mother will appear, to some degree, in the milk; but the quantity is usually less than 1% of the amount taken by the mother, and therefore has no harmful effect on the baby. Consider the following before taking medication during breastfeeding:

1. Will the medicine harm the baby?
2. Will the drug diminish milk production and thus indirectly harm the baby?
3. Do you really need the medication or could you handle your illness (e.g., a cold) without it?

While there are only a handful of drugs that absolutely cannot be taken while breastfeeding, our knowledge of the adverse effects of some medications is far from complete because it is difficult to measure the effects on the baby of medications present in breast milk.

The general advice when it comes to medicine is, "When in doubt, just say no." If a physician does not know whether or not a drug is safe, he will usually advise the patient not to breastfeed. Most pharmaceutical companies legally protect themselves with package inserts that advise a mother not to breastfeed while taking the drug. Unfortunately, we have seen babies weaned prematurely, abruptly and unnecessarily because of erroneous advice given about a harmless medication. Drug exposure to the nursing infant may be minimized by having the mother take the medication just after completing a breastfeeding and/or just before the infant has his lengthy sleep periods. Because most medications enter the milk within a few hours after ingestion, if the safety of the medication is uncertain and mother does not want to wean, she can pump both breasts and discard the milk for the next feeding after ingesting the medication. The following medications can be taken safely while breastfeeding:

DRUG	COMMENTS
Acetaminophen: Tylenol, Tempra, Panadol, Liquiprin	Safe while breastfeeding
Allergy medications: Antihistamines, decongestants	Most are safe. May cause sedation or hyperexcitability in infant, may occasionally decrease milk supply. Avoid long-acting preparations unless advised by physician.
Antacids	Safe
Antibiotics	Nearly all are safe to take during breastfeeding.
Keflex (cephalosporins)	Not excreted in milk, safest for infant; a good antibiotic for breast infections

Penicillin, Erythromycin, Furandantin	Safe
Flagyl	Not safe
Sulfa	Not safe in the newborn period (first four weeks); may produce jaundice in infant
Tetracycline	Not recommended for more than 10 days' use because may stain baby's teeth
Anticoagulants: Heparin, Warfarin	Heparin does not pass into breast milk. Warfarin has been studied and found to be safe.
Anticonvulsants	With physician's supervision.
Antidiarrheals	Safe
Antihypertensives	Safe
Aspirin	Safe if taken occasionally. Not safe to take in large amounts over a long period of time. Should not be taken without physician's advice; safer to use acetaminophen if possible.
Asthma medicines: Theophylline, Cromolyn, Albuterol	Safe if used under physician's supervision. Cromolyn has no harmful effect on infant.
Barium	Not absorbed—safe.
Chloroquine (antimalarial)	No harmful effect on infant.
Digitalis	Safe
Diuretics	Safe

Insulin	Safe
Isoniazid (tuberculosis drug)	Safe
Kaopectate	Safe
Laxatives	Some (e.g., Senakot and other senna preparations) may cause diarrhea or colic in infant.
Local anesthetics, e.g., those used for dental work	Safe
Narcotics:	
Codeine	Safe if used in small doses as a painkiller and only with physician's advice and supervision. Large and continued doses may depress or excite infant.
Morphine	Safe for single dose only and under medical supervision.
Cocaine and heroin	Not safe to take during breastfeeding.
Pinworm medication	Safe
Propanolol	Safe
Sedatives: Barbiturates, Valium, and chloralhydrate	Safe if taken under physician's supervision. Too high a dosage for too long a time can depress or excite infant. Valium should not be used in the first postpartum week.
Thyroid medication	Thyroid supplement medication is safe if used under physician's supervision. Some drugs to suppress thyroid function are unsafe

	during breastfeeding; consult your physician concerning the specific antithyroid medication.
Tranquilizers	Many are safe, some are not; must check with physician. Most in large doses and over a long period of time may cause drowsiness and poor feeding in infants and are therefore not recommended.
Vaccines	Safe
Vitamins	Safe

- Nearly all over-the-counter medications are safe in a single or even a daily dose, but it is wise to check with your doctor.
- Take any medication immediately after breastfeeding so your system will have as much time as possible to break down the drug before baby's next feeding.
- If you must take a potentially harmful medication, you do not need to permanently wean your baby. You can express or pump and discard your milk while on the medication and resume nursing when the medication is no longer in your system. Most medications are safely cleared from your system within 48 hours after discontinuing; check with your doctor on this.
- The age of your baby is important. Generally, the older the infant, the safer the medication taken during breastfeeding. Newborns have a limited ability to handle most medications; consider this the highest-risk period for taking medicines while breastfeeding. The effects of a drug on your infant may be unpredictable, so keep an eye on him. Consult your doctor about which symptoms to watch for in the baby; the

usual warning signs of a harmful drug effect are vomiting, diarrhea, lethargy, jaundice, poor feeding, fast heart rate, unusual crying, and irritability.

DRUGS THAT ARE CONTRAINDICATED DURING BREASTFEEDING

- Amphetamines
- Antimetabolite drugs (anticancer drugs)
- Antithyroid (some)
- Cocaine
- Cyclosporin
- Ergotamine
- Flagyl
- Heroin
- Lithium
- Marijuana
- Methotrexate
- Mysoline
- Nicotine
- Parlodel
- PCP
- Radioactive iodides

Radioactive Drugs for Diagnostic Procedures

A breastfeeding mother may need to have a diagnostic procedure requiring her to take a radioactive drug. This radioactivity would enter her breast milk and ultimately her baby. Take the following precautionary steps if you need to take a radioactive drug:

- Be sure you absolutely need this procedure at this time. Can it be delayed until after weaning?
- Consult a nuclear medicine specialist and request a drug that clears from your breast milk most quickly. The three radioactive diagnostic drugs that are commonly used in radiologic tests are gallium, iodine, and technetium.

- Depending on the type of radioactive drug used, breastfeeding should be discontinued for 24 to 72 hours, during which time the mother should continue to pump her breasts and discard the milk.

Oral Contraceptives and Breastfeeding

Studies in mothers taking the older oral contraceptive pill (containing both estrogen and progestin) show that it causes a decrease in the quality and quantity of breast milk and that small amounts of the hormones enter the milk. The infants of these mothers show slower weight gain. The long-term effects of an infant's exposure to these hormones is not yet known. For these reasons, the combined estrogen/progestin pill is definitely not recommended for a breastfeeding mother. Whether or not the use of the minipill (progestin only) is safe during breastfeeding is still unresolved. Studies have shown no decrease in the quantity or quality of milk produced or of weight gain in the infants whose mothers have taken the minipill. (We have, however, talked with mothers who notice a drop in milk supply.) Because the long-term effects of the minipill on the infant are as yet unknown, most breastfeeding authorities recommend that no form of oral contraceptive be taken during breastfeeding, and that barrier methods or natural family planning be used if contraception is desired.

Environmental Contaminants

In the past decade there has been a flurry of attention about the contamination of breast milk by industrial chemicals, such as DDT, which was withdrawn from the market in 1972. Now pesticides and industrial chemicals that pollute the water are under scrutiny. These chemicals, which have an affinity for animal fat, tend to concentrate in breast milk because of its high fat content. Although the concern is justified, you should not decide against breastfeeding because of environmental contaminants.

Cases in which infants become sick because of environmental chemicals in breast milk are *very rare.* Most reported infant illnesses caused by breast milk contaminants have resulted from exposure to occupational chemicals during pregnancy and lactation. Since the benefits of breastfeeding far outweigh the risk of contaminants in breast milk, pregnant and lactating mothers should take the following steps to protect themselves and their babies from environmental pollutants:

1. Avoid occupations in which you work in close contact with hazardous chemicals during pregnancy and lactation.
2. Avoid eating fish from waters known to be contaminated with industrial chemicals.
3. If pesticide contamination is suspected, fruits and vegetables should be peeled and washed thoroughly.
4. Avoid excess weight loss during lactation. This may mobilize the chemicals from fats stored in your breast milk.

Because information concerning drugs and breast milk is constantly being updated, if your physician is uncertain whether or not a medication you must take is safe during breastfeeding, consult a local lactation specialist or call the La Leche League.

References:

1. "Transfer of drugs and other chemicals into human milk," Committee on Drugs, The American Academy of Pediatrics, *Pediatrics,* Vol. 84, 1989.

2. *Breastfeeding—A Guide for the Medical Profession* by Ruth Lawrence, M.D., 1989. The Mosby Company, St. Louis.
3. *Drugs in Pregnancy and Lactation: A Reference Guide to Fetal and Neonatal Risk.* Third edition. Briggs, Freeman, Yaffe. 1990. Williams & Wilkins, Baltimore.

32

SMOKING AND SECOND-HAND SMOKE

Smoking is definitely to be avoided because of its detrimental effects on both mother and baby. It has recently been discovered that smoking may reduce a mother's prolactin level. Not only do mothers need prolactin to make sufficient milk but they need this hormone to offer sufficient mothering. The last thing a mother wants to do is take a drug (which is what nicotine is) that lowers her mothering skills and decreases her milk supply. Studies have also shown that smoking may interfere with the milk ejection reflex. Nicotine passes through your milk to the baby; its effects on the baby are unknown.

The passive effects of second-hand smoke are especially harmful to the baby. When you smoke, your baby smokes. During pregnancy this is certainly true but in a different mechanism—the nicotine from your blood passes directly to the baby. Baby's tiny nasal passages are exquisitely sensitive to cigarette smoke, leading to stuffy noses, respiratory infections and consequent difficulty breastfeeding. If you simply cannot kick the habit of smoking completely, at least try to minimize the number of cigarettes you smoke each day and *certainly do not smoke around baby.* One study showed that the incidence of colic was 50% higher in infants of breastfeeding mothers who smoked. It would also be wise for mothers to insist that nobody smoke in the house, car, or room that baby is in, as this may upset his sensitive breathing passages.

33

ALCOHOL AND RECREATIONAL DRUGS

Alcohol and breastfeeding. Breastfeeding folklore has traditionally encouraged an occasional glass of wine to relax the mother, and has preached that "Beer is good for increasing milk supply." New research calls into question the advice given to some new mothers that they have a drink to relax during breastfeeding. A recent study published in *The New England Journal of Medicine* found that the one-year-old children of women who had one to four drinks a day (a drink was defined as one bottle of beer, one glass of wine or one cocktail) scored slightly lower on motor-skill tests but showed no difference in mental tests, compared to mothers who had less than one drink. Though it has been repeated by other researchers, the study cautioned that these results were too preliminary to draw any definite conclusions.

A safe level of alcohol consumption for breastfeeding women has not been determined, but we do know that alcohol ingested during breastfeeding enters the bloodstream and quickly migrates to the milk. Researchers theorize that the infant brain may be exquisitely sensitive to small quantities of pure alcohol; or the infant may be unable to metabolize alcohol as quickly as an adult, so it accumulates in the child's body. There is general agreement that a large amount of alcohol consumed over a long period of time by the breastfeeding mother may harm her infant's development. As is true of most drugs, what is not known is the minimum level of alcohol that a mother can consume without harming the infant at all. At this writing, breastfeeding consultants are comfortable with advising a mother that one or two drinks per week should not harm her baby. Because the topic of alcohol consumption while breastfeeding is so important, I advise mothers to check with their physician or lactation consultant about the latest research in this matter.

What about recreational drugs such as marijuana? Like alcohol, the research on the effects of marijuana on the breastfeeding infant is still inconclusive. Studies with laboratory animals have shown structural changes in the brain cells of the nursing animals after their mothers were exposed to marijuana. Marijuana has been found to lower the levels of prolactin in the mother, and THC, the active chemical in marijuana, appears in breast milk in small amounts. These experimental effects plus the possible effect of marijuana on lowering a mother's attentiveness to her baby should dictate, by common sense, that mothers avoid marijuana during breastfeeding.

Cocaine, a more powerful and more dangerous drug, enters the milk of the breastfeeding mother and may stimulate the baby's nervous system, causing colicky symptoms, irritability and sleeplessness. This drug should definitely be avoided. Depressant drugs such as heroin should also obviously be avoided.

34

BREASTFEEDING AS A NATURAL CONTRACEPTIVE

Does breastfeeding really work as a natural contraceptive? Yes!—as long as the rules of the game are followed. Studies in our culture and others have shown that breastfeeding can inhibit fertility for an average of 14.6 months in mothers who follow certain rules when using breastfeeding as a natural contraceptive. Studies comparing breastfeeding according to the rules and "Western-style" breastfeeding (which means less frequent feeding, less nighttime feeding and using pacifiers and supplements) showed that lactational amenorrhea (infertility induced by breastfeeding) averaged 13 to 14 months in the first group and 8 to 9 months in the second.

The rules of the game. Breastfeeding is at least 95% effective as a child spacing method as long as the following practices are followed:

- Unrestricted breastfeeding without regard to daytime or nighttime scheduling.
- Unrestricted night nursing, preferably with mother and baby sleeping together.
- Artificial feeding delayed until at least six months. Solid foods should not substitute for breastfeeding but rather add to baby's overall food intake.
- Pacifiers or supplemental bottles should not be used.

Here's how this beautiful natural system of child spacing works. Baby's sucking on the nipple stimulates production of the mothering hormone, prolactin. The high level of circulating prolactin in the mother's blood suppresses the levels of estrogen and progesterone, the hormones that are necessary for ovulation and the preparation of the womb for implantation of a fertilized egg. When ovulation does not occur and there are no changes in the lining of the uterus, the mother is infertile and does not have menstrual periods. As the frequency of breastfeeding lessens and baby is given alternate methods of nutrition and comfort, the baby sucks less often and mother's level of prolactin falls. Estrogen and progesterone levels rise and the first postpartum menstrual period occurs, a signal that a woman is or most likely will be fertile again. Shortly after this "warning menses," ovulation resumes and fertility returns. The amount of sucking stimulation and the level of prolactin required to suppress these reproductive hormones vary from woman to woman; but in general, frequent and intense sucking is required to suppress ovulation.

Frequent breastfeeding is the number-one stimulus for maintaining high prolactin levels. Mothers who remain infertile the longest during lactation breastfeed the longest, suckle their babies more frequently, maintain night nursing, and introduce supplemental feedings the latest and the most gradually, when compared with mothers who practice more Western-style parenting. In some studies, ovulation returned to mothers when they breastfed less than six times per day and the total duration of sucking was less than 60 minutes a day.

The suppression of ovulation and menstruation depends upon a consistently high level of prolactin in the mother's blood. Because prolactin has a short half-life (meaning that it dissipates rapidly from the blood), frequent stimulation of prolactin production is necessary to maintain this consistently high level and suppress fertility. Studies have shown that when artificial feedings were substituted for breastfeedings rather than being used as an occasional complement to breastfeeding, mothers showed a diminishing prolactin level.

Prolactin levels are also dependent on nighttime feedings. When babies in a study began to sleep through feedings more often, there was a decrease in mothers' prolactin levels. It has also been shown that when babies "sleep through the night" mothers will soon resume menstruation.

Why does this natural method of child-spacing work so well in other countries and not the Western world? The main reason is the difference in nighttime parenting styles. Prolactin is highest during sleep. Western mothers often try to bunch up the day feedings and space out night feedings in hopes of getting baby to "sleep through the night." Cultures in which this contraceptive system works offer more unrestricted night nursing.

One of the most highly studied cultures is the !Kung tribe, a hunting and gathering people in Africa. In this culture, the infants are always in immediate physical proximity to the mother until two years of age or older. Babies sleep on the same skin mat with mother until weaned, and mother and baby enjoy unrestricted night nursing. When questioned about night nursing, mothers respond that their infants "nursed many times" throughout the night without waking. The babies nurse in short, frequent bouts throughout the day and as often as several times per hour. Among the mothers of this culture, the average birth interval is 44 months. No other forms of contraception are used and there are no taboos on sexual intercourse during lactation. Smaller studies on a group of mothers practicing this parenting style in Western cultures have yielded similar results.

The return of menses following childbirth usually occurs before ovulation and serves as a warning that fertility may soon resume. In a small percentage of lactating women (less than 5%), ovulation occurs before the first menses, and the mother may not know that her fertility has returned. Ovulation occurring before the first menses is more likely to happen toward the end of breastfeeding, that is, after the baby is a year old. Because the absence of menstrual periods is not an infallible indication of infertility, it is wise for breastfeeding mothers to know about other signs of returning fertility. Women throughout history have learned to read their natural body processes to determine when they are fertile. Changes in the amount and type of cervical mucus are one of the signs to indicate imminent ovulation. There are many classes on natural family planning techniques that help a mother learn her body's individual fertility signs. One of the most complete references on the subject of breastfeeding as a natural contraceptive is *Breastfeeding and Natural Child Spacing* by Sheila Kippley (Penguin Books, New York, 1989).

Parents who are "blessed" with an infant who schedules easily, spaces feedings easily, sleeps through the night and wants early solids are also more likely to be blessed with children who are close in age.

35

BREASTFEEDING WHILE PREGNANT

There is a lot of misinformation about whether it is safe to breastfeed one baby while pregnant with another. Many obstetricians caution mothers not to breastfeed during pregnancy. Here is the reason *in theory.* Breastfeeding stimulates the hormone oxytocin to be secreted into your bloodstream. This hormone acts on the uterus to stimulate contractions, possibly inducing a miscarriage. In actual experience this doesn't happen. We have interviewed obstetricians who are knowledgeable about the mother's hormonal system during pregnancy. It seems that the uterus is not receptive to the hormonal stimulation from oxytocin until around 24 weeks of gestation, so it is safe for a mother to breastfeed at least until around 20 weeks. Current evidence, then, suggests that breastfeeding during pregnancy is indeed safe, unless a risk of preterm labor develops.

Many mothers successfully breastfeed during some or all of their pregnancy without doing any harm to mother or baby. If you have a history of miscarriages or if you experience uterine contractions during breastfeeding, consult your obstetrician; it may be wise to stop. It is best to check with your doctor about whether it is safe to breastfeed during your particular pregnancy.

Most mothers experience exquisite nipple tenderness during pregnancy, making breastfeeding uncomfortable. Also expect your milk to change in taste during the final three months of pregnancy; it is common for a nursing toddler to give a "don't like anymore" signal during this time, and to self-wean. A diminished milk supply is also typical during pregnancy. If you have a baby under the age of one who still relies heavily on breast milk for his nourishment, you may need to supplement with more solid food or even some formula.

Pregnancy is a time of natural weaning for many babies due to the changes in the character and quantity of the breast milk. And nipple sensitivity motivates many mothers who would otherwise welcome a longer breastfeeding relationship to encourage the baby to cut down considerably on his time at breast.

If your baby is highly attached to breastfeeding and seems unready to be completely weaned, consider continuing to breastfeed at a level that you can handle. Negotiate shorter times at the breast and limit the nursing times to, perhaps, just nap- and bedtime, or whenever suits the two of you. One important advantage of breastfeeding through a pregnancy is that the arrival of a new baby is less threatening when the older one still has his place at the breast. Families who have experienced this sharing at the breast say that sibling rivalry is greatly reduced.

36

BREASTFEEDING THE ADOPTED BABY

Over the past 20 years we have counseled many adoptive mothers in the art and science of breastfeeding their adopted babies. Like any good investment, the initial price may be high but the returns are great.

How much do you really want to breastfeed? Intellectually you may have heard and read that breastfeeding is best for your baby physically and emotionally. But are you emotionally prepared for the time, energy and commitment you will need to get your milk flowing? This is called "induced lactation," meaning that certain techniques are used to get your milk flowing, since the adoptive mother will not initially have the hormones of pregnancy to get the milk-producing system started. Even pregnant mothers need to work at breastfeeding a bit, though their hormones have naturally initiated the process. An adoptive mother will have to work at it much more.

Seek advice and support from mothers who have successfully breastfed their adoptive babies. A list of women in your area can be obtained by contacting your local La Leche League or a lactation consultant in your area.

Consult a lactation specialist as soon as you know that you will be adopting a baby. If you are blessed with the ideal situation—that is, hearing about your baby before it is born—begin inducing lactation around a month before baby's anticipated birth. Rent an electric breast pump, preferably one with a double pumping system, and simulate breastfeeding by pumping your breasts as often as you would feed your newborn, around every three hours. Your lactation specialist will show you how to use the pump and to gradually build up the time and frequency of pumping.

The next step in the continuum of breastfeeding the adoptive baby is to make arrangements with the obstetrician ahead of time to either be present at the delivery or to bond with your baby shortly after the birth. It is necessary for the baby to know as quickly as possible to whom he or she belongs. It would also be wise for you to begin the first feedings before baby gets confused with artificial nipples. Because you will have little (or none) of your own milk right after birth, this feeding is done by the use of an ingenious device called an S.N.S. (supplemental nutrition system—see Key 20), which simulates breastfeeding. The lactation specialist will also show you how to position and latch baby on properly to your breast so that he or she learns to suck.

The key to breastfeeding the adopted baby is to simulate, as much as possible, the natural biological techniques of breastfeeding. Try to be present for as many feedings as you can while baby is in the hospital. Since you may not be able to be present for all of them, instruct the nurses to use the finger and syringe method of feeding or to let baby use the nursing supplementer and suck from the nurse's finger. In this technique the tubing from the supplementer is placed along the tip of the nurse's finger, so that when baby sucks on her finger he also gets milk from the tubing. Again, try to avoid unnecessary bottle feeding in the early days and weeks that baby is learning to adapt to this supplemental nutrition system. The more the baby is given his feedings at your breast, the more stimulation you have for producing your own milk.

In the early days of inducing lactation with your new baby, remember that it is frequent sucking that will bring your milk in. Nurse baby as often as your energy and baby's temperament permit, using the nursing supplementer at as many feedings as you can. The more baby sucks from your breast, the more he induces your own milk-producing systems to click in. Over the ensuing weeks you will begin to produce milk. We caution adoptive breastfeeding mothers not to be too focused on how soon and how much they will produce. Few mothers ever produce a quantity or quality of milk that will totally satisfy baby, and it is realistic to be prepared to need some supplemental formula. The whole act of breastfeeding and the close bonding it entails are what is important.

Many adoptive mothers achieve some degree of their own milk production within a couple of weeks after beginning to breastfeed. If a mother has previously given birth and/or has breastfed previous babies, she is likely to produce more milk. Other methods to help increase milk supply are massaging before feedings, sleeping with the baby and allowing unrestricted night nursing.

Not only is breastfeeding good for the adopted baby, it does good things for mother too. Every time your baby sucks from your nipple, he stimulates the flow of the milk-producing hormone prolactin, also called the "mothering hormone" because it is thought to stimulate mothering instincts. Breastfeeding an adopted baby is a classic example of the saying, "Where there's a will there's a way."

37

BREASTFEEDING THE JAUNDICED BABY

Most newborns develop some degree of jaundice (yellow color of the skin and eyeballs). Jaundice is caused by a buildup in the blood of a yellow pigment called bilirubin, and the deposit of the excess bilirubin in the skin. Everyone normally produces some bilirubin from the breakdown of old, worn-out red blood cells (newborns produce more bilirubin because their red blood cells break down more quickly than those of adults). This bilirubin is usually disposed of by the liver and therefore does not normally reach high enough levels to yellow the skin. But if too many red blood cells are broken down too fast or if the liver is unable to remove the bilirubin from the blood, the visual appearance of jaundice results.

Newborns are susceptible to two types of jaundice, normal and abnormal. We use the term "normal" jaundice (also called physiologic jaundice) because many babies have it to some degree; "normal" jaundice is thought to be due to temporary immaturity of the liver. Within a few days, the liver matures and begins disposing of the excess bilirubin. Your pediatrician will tell you whether your baby's jaundice is normal; if it is, there's no need for worry. Normal jaundice is a source of much unnecessary anxiety at a time when a new breastfeeding mother is very vulnerable to any suggestion that her baby might be abnormal. It is important that the attending medical personnel not present normal jaundice as an illness, for anything that causes mother anxiety can diminish the very hormones that are needed to make milk.

It is very rarely necessary to temporarily stop breastfeeding if a baby has this *normal* type of jaundice. The reason for the unwarranted scare about breastfeeding causing jaundice is due to a very rare condition (probably accounting for no more than 1% of jaundiced babies) in which breast milk can aggravate jaundice. The mechanism of this is still unknown but it is thought to be due to a temporary substance in breast milk that prolongs the normal physiologic jaundice. The criteria for the diagnosis of "breast milk jaundice" are: it begins after the fourth day of life; and the bilirubin count diminishes by 4 milligrams after breastfeeding is discontinued for 24 hours. The implication that breastfeeding may aggravate *all* types of jaundice has unfortunately led to many mothers being advised to stop breastfeeding temporarily if their babies develop jaundice.

Experts who have studied the correlation between breastfeeding and jaundice believe that it is rarely necessary for a mother to stop breastfeeding if her baby has normal physiologic jaundice. Picture the following scenario: baby has normal physiologic jaundice and mother is advised to stop breastfeeding. Baby is then separated from the mother and put under a phototherapy lamp (special lights that dissolve the bilirubin in the skin, allowing it to be excreted in the urine and reducing the bilirubin level). The separation from the mother during phototherapy time, in addition to the fact that phototherapy makes babies sleepy and somewhat dehydrated, makes some babies disinterested in breastfeeding. This lack of interest combined with the separation from mother leads to diminished milk supply at a vulnerable time when frequent sucking and continued presence of the baby is necessary to stimulate mother's milk. Because her milk does not appear mother feels like a failure and does not enjoy breastfeeding—and another "breastfeeding failure" unfortunately occurs.

None of this should happen. If your baby is jaundiced, be sure the medical personnel are up to date on the fact that it is very rarely necessary to separate a breastfeeding mother from her jaundiced baby. Even if phototherapy is necessary (and it usually is not with normal jaundice), there are phototherapy lights now available that are incorporated into the baby's blanket and wrapped around him. Mother can then hold and breastfeed baby while he is receiving phototherapy.

In fact, a breastfeeding mother can lessen the degree of jaundice in her baby by rooming-in with the baby. Rooming-in infants nurse more often, get more milk and mother's milk is established sooner. Because the milk washes out the meconium in the intestines, and also the excess bilirubin, the more breast milk baby gets the less jaundiced he will become.

If your baby has abnormal-type jaundice requiring phototherapy, expect him to become very sleepy and temporarily uninterested in breastfeeding. If this happens, consult a lactation specialist for special ways of stimulating his interest. Undress him, promoting skin-to-skin contact. Use your nipple to stimulate baby's lips, and allow him to suck in continuous bursts and pauses. Baby will suck a little and snooze a little, suck a little and snooze a little. You will be surprised how much milk even a sleepy baby will get, because it is the frequency of nursing that is more important than the intensity. If baby is truly not getting enough breast milk due to sleepiness or frustration, he should be supplemented with pumped breast milk, not with formula. This extra breast milk should be fed by medicine cup, dropper or syringe, avoiding the use of bottle and nipple, which can cause nipple confusion.

You should be able to breastfeed your baby even in cases of abnormal jaundice caused by a problem such as a blood group incompatibility. Discuss with your doctor the safety and benefits of breastfeeding your jaundiced baby.

38

BREASTFEEDING TWINS

Breastfeeding twins requires twice the commitment, twice the energy and twice the sense of humor—but the returns on your investment are also doubled. Even singleton babies nurse frequently during the day and sometimes also during the night. Double that with twins.

To both survive and thrive with breastfeeding twins, try the following tips:

- **Get the right start.** Most twins are premature, which adds an extra challenge to breastfeeding. Because prematures tend to be sleepy and to have a weak suck for a couple of weeks, it is very important to seek help from a lactation consultant within a day or two after birth. Efficient milk delivery is the key to breastfeeding twins. For this reason, learn proper positioning and latch-on techniques immediately before your nipples get sore, your milk becomes insufficient and the babies learn poor sucking habits. Right start techniques are important enough for single babies; they are doubly important to learn for twins.
- **Nurse separately, then simultaneously.** Early on as babies are learning to suck properly, most mothers find it easier to nurse one baby at a time, devoting her full attention to each so they learn proper latch-on. Once babies have learned to latch on correctly, simultaneous nursing for most feedings will be easier for you. Most mothers of twins try to feed simultaneously for most of the feedings and individually once or twice a day so that each one gets some individual attention. This will most likely happen when one

twin is hungry and the other is asleep. If both babies have similar temperaments and feeding needs, simultaneous nursing is easier.

Sometimes one is a high-need baby and the other is easy, and one is hungrier than the other. It is best to let the hungrier and more frequent nurser set the pattern; as you are about to feed the hungrier baby, wake the other one for a feeding also. Simultaneous nursing also implies getting babies onto a similar sleep schedule.

- **Position for nursing twins.** There are three positions for simultaneously nursing twins:

  1. *The clutch hold* (also called the football position. Place both babies on pillows under your arms and nurse simultaneously). This position allows you to control their head movements more easily in case one or both tend to be archers, throwing their heads back during nursing.
  2. *Criss-crossed position.* Babies are criss-crossed across their mother's tummy and mother holds each one across the back, clasping her hands under their buttocks. Mother's arms are each supported by pillows under the elbows and perhaps another pillow on her lap.
  3. *Babies are placed facing the same direction*, unlike that of the criss-cross direction. In the criss-cross direction the baby who nurses from the right breast has his feet pointing toward the left side and vice versa. In the same-direction nursing position, both babies' feet stretch toward the same side. Again, pillows under the arms and in the lap are a must. A footstool is also an absolute must for nursing twins in order to better elevate your lap and contain both babies.

- **Scheduling twins.** It is better to alternate breasts, since most mothers find that one breast will produce more milk than the other and babies will soon develop a breast preference. As for a schedule, whatever works is the right one for you. Simultaneous nursing and similar sleep schedules are ideal if it works. In the early months most twins will sleep better side by side in the same crib or cradle; after all, they have been "womb mates" for nine months. After six months, when babies get somewhat restless, they often wake each other, necessitating separate sleeping arrangements.
- **Get dad involved.** In fact, father involvement in breastfeeding twins is not a request, it is an absolute necessity. The mother-father roles are not so well defined in parenting twins. It is true that only mother can make milk, but dad can do everything else. Mothers who have successfully breastfed twins have mastered the art of delegating household responsibilities to their husband. This is especially true if supplemental bottles are given (and they frequently are needed)—the babies get only breast milk from mother and formula by bottle from dad. One father of twins in our practice summed up this shared parenting with, "Our babies have two mothers; she is the milk mother and I am the other mother." By this he meant that mother breastfeeds but he does everything else around the house, so that she can save her energy to do what she does best. Fatigue is what does most breastfeeding mothers in. Fathers play a very crucial role in minimizing this fatigue.

Most mothers of twins describe the first year as a "blur," meaning that they are often so tired that they function somewhat mechanically, at times not remembering what they did even though they managed to do it. The constant-maintenance stage of breastfeeding twins will soon pass and you will reap many benefits of the hours you spent in this special relationship with both of your babies. It is worth it!

Helpful resources for breastfeeding twins:
National Organization of Mothers of Twins Club,
5402 Amberwood Lane,
Rockville, MD 20853
(301) 460-9108.

Reprint on breastfeeding twins available from La Leche League.

39

BREASTFEEDING SPECIAL BABIES IN SPECIAL CIRCUMSTANCES

A special kind of parenting is necessary for special babies. If you have a baby with special needs, breastfeeding is even more important. It is important for you because of the added hormonal stimulation breastfeeding provides to give you a higher level of prolactin. It is important for baby because of the physical, medical, and psychological benefits that breastfeeding provides.

Breastfeeding the baby with Down syndrome (and other babies with hypotonia). Because babies with Down syndrome are more prone to respiratory infections (especially ear infections), the extra immunity to germs provided by breast milk is very important to these babies. Down syndrome babies are also prone to intestinal infections. Breast milk contains substances that promote the growth of friendly bacteria in the intestinal tract, a factor which lessens intestinal infections.

Here is another reason that mothers have shared with us why they have persevered in breastfeeding their Down syndrome babies. Breast milk contains taurine, an amino acid that promotes brain growth. These mothers stated that they want to do everything possible to help their special baby reach his or her potential. Some Down syndrome babies have a heart problem that causes them to tire more easily during feedings. Recent research with premature and sick newborns has shown that a breastfeeding baby sucks in short bursts and pauses, actually spending less energy during a feeding than a bottle-fed baby does. The low salt content of human milk is better for a baby with heart problems. With these benefits in mind, here are some helpful tips on successfully breastfeeding your baby with Down syndrome.

- **Get the right start.** Because these babies have a weak musculature, their sucking mechanism, especially their tongue action, is also weak. These babies need to be trained to suck efficiently. Some babies with normal muscle tone can suck incorrectly and get by with it; a Down syndrome baby cannot. They must be taught proper latch-on techniques. And some Down babies do have a very strong suck, so proper latch-on will prevent sore nipples. Consult a lactation specialist or visit a breastfeeding center with experience in breastfeeding Down babies. Special exercises are needed to teach the baby to open his mouth wider and curl his tongue properly, and to teach mother how to position the nipple and areola far into the baby's mouth to stimulate proper latch-on. This consultation should be done within the first few days. These babies frequently need to be supplemented during the first days and weeks as they are learning to suck properly. Above all do not use a bottle because this will teach them lazy sucking habits. If supplementary milk is necessary, pump your breast milk and supplement the breastfeeding with a medicine dropper, syringe or nursing supplementer. Specific breastfeeding helps for Down syndrome babies are:
  - Give extra support to baby's head during the first three months, as these babies have weak neck muscles and are unable to support their own heads.

- Press down on your baby's chin to encourage baby to open his mouth widely.
- The Down syndrome baby has a somewhat thick, flat tongue that is initially unable to cup around the nipple and form a groove that carries milk to the back of the throat. By pressing down on the center of the tongue with a finger several times before each feeding, the mother can help her baby learn to shape his tongue correctly.
- Get used to pressing down on your baby's tongue with your finger as a normal exercise between feedings so that baby learns to cup his tongue and place it underneath your nipple. Sometimes baby's tongue will elevate above the nipple and actually keep the milk from entering the back of the mouth.
- Because Down syndrome babies are generally easy and nondemanding, you will have to initiate the feeding schedule. Most of these babies simply do not demand to be fed as often as they need it. Feed every two hours by day and every three hours at night.
- Some mothers have a very active milk ejection reflex, causing large volumes of milk to squirt out during a feeding. These babies often cannot handle the onslaught of extra milk and begin to gag. As soon as you notice your milk spurting out too fast, release baby from the breast, waste a few spurts and put your baby back on. As he gets older and develops a more coordinated suck-swallow mechanism, the baby will adjust to the increased flow of milk.
- Wear your baby in a baby sling as much as possible. Proximity to mother stimulates feeding frequency, and Down syndrome babies need to be fed more frequently.
- The added touch, eye contact, stroking and overall stimulation that the whole interaction of breastfeeding provides is especially important for these special babies.

The following are resources for breastfeeding the baby with Down syndrome:
The reprint, "Breastfeeding the Baby with Down Syndrome," available from La Leche League.
National Down Syndrome Congress,
1800 Dempster, Park Ridge, IL 60068-1146,
(1-800) 232-6372, In Illinois (312) 823-7550.
National Association for Down Syndrome,
P.O. Box 4542, Oak Brook, IL 60521,
(312) 325-9112.
Mother and Infant Services,
6201 Middle Fiskville, Suite C-3, Austin, TX 78750,
(512) 836-3456.

Breastfeeding the baby with cleft lip and/or palate. Babies with a cleft lip or palate present another challenge to breastfeeding. As in babies with Down syndrome, these babies are also prone to ear infections, primarily because of the regurgitation of milk into the eustachean tubes positioned above the cleft in the palate. Theoretically any foreign milk (formula or cow's milk) can irritate the eustachean tube more than human milk, so here again breast milk should lower the incidence of ear infections in these babies.

Because of the cleft in the lip and palate, these babies are not able to create a suction to draw the nipple far enough into the mouth and compress the nipple and areola between tongue below and palate above. Within the first couple of days, obtain help from a certified lactation consultant or from a breastfeeding center with experience in feeding babies with this condition. A specialist will show you how to position your baby so that he will not choke during feedings. Babies should be fed in a semi-upright position and have small, frequent feedings; mother will learn when to interrupt the feedings as baby begins to get too much milk leaking up through the nose. As baby is learning how to suck properly from the breast it is often necessary to supplement using a syringe or nursing supplementer. Pump your breasts after each feeding and supplement your baby with your own milk.

Breastfeeding specialists have actually found that suction plays a very minor part in drawing milk from the breast. It is the coordinated action of the tongue, cheeks, jaws, and gums that extrudes milk from the breast. Teaching all of these oral parts to function properly is what a lactation consultant can do. The suction provided during breastfeeding is mainly to keep mother's nipple in baby's mouth. Mother can be taught how to do this for the baby. Surgical repair of cleft lips and palate is being done earlier and earlier, so you are simply temporizing during those early months until surgical repair of the cleft is performed. During the temporary weaning for surgical repair, remember to pump your breast to keep up your milk supply.

The baby with congenital heart disease. Babies who are born with certain heart defects have one or the other of the following problems: they either have too much blood flowing to their lungs, causing overload on the heart, or they have insufficient blood flow to the lungs, resulting in blueness (cyanosis). Both of these conditions cause baby to be extremely tired during feedings. Years ago it was erroneously thought that breastfeeding would tire these babies out too much; recent evidence shows the opposite to be true. The breastfeeding baby sucks in short bursts and pauses, resting frequently between sucking. Premature and sick newborn babies have been shown to lose less energy and to breathe more effectively during breastfeeding than bottle feeding. The lower salt content in breast milk is also more beneficial to babies who are prone to heart failure. In light of this new information, most newborn centers are encouraging mothers to breastfeed premature babies, newborns with breathing difficulties, and babies with congenital heart disease. But special breastfeeding help is still needed for these special babies. An initial nursing supplementer is often necessary, using your pumped breast milk in a syringe or other supplementer while the baby is learning to suck more efficiently. Smaller, shorter, more frequent feedings are necessary in babies with congenital heart disease. Each year there is more and more research showing the therapeutic value of human milk for human babies—and their parents.

Special Circumstances for Parents

Tandem nursing means nursing a new baby and an older sibling. Most toddlers will wean (or their mothers want them to) during pregnancy with another baby. Some toddlers, however, enjoy this beautiful relationship and do not want to give it up, nor do their mothers. Tandem nursing is possible, though tiring.

Most mothers have ambivalent feelings about tandem nursing. On the one hand, they do not want to deprive the older child of a special relationship if they truly feel this child is not ready to be weaned. On the other hand, most mothers find this practice too draining. We encourage mothers who consider tandem nursing to remember that the younger baby needs your milk; the older baby wants your milk. We have found it helpful to "deal" with the older sibling, such as, "We only nurse when the sun goes down and when the sun comes up." Nursing down to sleep and nursing in the morning are the two favorite times of day for a toddler. Sometimes the older toddler will simply want to nurse during high-need periods such as an illness, or will want a frequent pick-me-up of one- or two-minute nursings, and then they are off in their busy little world. This stage will soon pass as you and your husband learn alternative ways to distract your toddler and channel his or her interest in a direction away from the breast.

Your older sibling is only a toddler for a very short time and this nursing stage will soon pass.

Breastfeeding following breast surgery. Most procedures for breast enlargement (augmentation mammoplasty) do not harm the milk ducts and should not interfere with breastfeeding. Depending on how the procedure was performed, an occasional mother may report diminished milk supply and need to supplement the baby. In this circumstance the use of a supplementer may be necessary.

Breast reduction (reduction mammoplasty), on the other hand, quite often interferes with sufficient milk supply because of the more extensive surgery that is needed and the risk of damage to milk ducts. Unless medically indicated, it is wise to wait until after your childbearing years to undergo this procedure. If it is medically indicated, you can still breastfeed but supplementation will probably be necessary.

Breastfeeding while mother is ill. As discussed in Key 31, nearly all medications taken for common illnesses such as flu and sore throat are safe to take while breastfeeding. In most instances it is completely safe to breastfeed your baby during common illnesses. The most common one we encounter is intestinal flu causing vomiting and diarrhea in the mother. But breast milk actually protects baby against many of these germs, because when a mother's body harbors a germ she produces antibodies to it. The antibodies in her blood enter her breast milk and are transferred to her baby, thus immunizing him against it. The most common problem in breastfeeding while ill is dehydration due to vomiting and/or diarrhea, which may temporarily diminish your milk supply. To prevent this from happening, drink a lot of extra fluids (try sucking on popsicles all day long) or the sips-and-chips method (sip small amounts of fluid frequently with ice chips).

40

WEANING: WHEN AND HOW

We have a sign in our breastfeeding center, "Early weaning not recommended for babies." There are more breastfeeding mothers today, and they are breastfeeding longer. While the time of weaning varies tremendously from baby to baby and according to each family's individual situation, let's examine what we believe is the ideal timing and method of weaning a baby (keeping in mind that the ideal is not always achievable).

We may gain some insight into the real meaning of the term "weaning" by examining what weaning meant in ancient times. In ancient writings the word "weaning" meant "to ripen"; it implied a readiness. Weaning did not mean a loss or detachment from a relationship, but rather a passage from one relationship to another. When a child was weaned it was a festive occasion, and not because of what you may think—"Now I can finally get away from this child. . . ." It was a joyous occasion because a weaned child was regarded as a fulfilled child, i.e., a child who was so trusting and secure that he was ready to wean from a relationship of being dependent on the mother into the more independent stages of childhood. A beautiful description of the significance of weaning is found in the writings of King David, "But I have stilled and quieted my soul, like a weaned child with its mother, like a weaned child is my soul within me." The psalmist, David, equates his feeling of peace and tranquility with the feeling a weaned child has from trusting its mother. In ancient times and in many cultures even today a baby is nursed for two or three *years* (or more). In Western culture we are accustomed to thinking of breastfeeding in terms of months. We would like to change this mindset.

When to wean? We have stressed throughout this book that some babies have higher and longer needs than others. This is why one should not set an arbitrary time limit on weaning a child. If a mother and father have practiced the attachment style of parenting from birth, they will intuitively know when and at what pace to wean their child. Some people may feel that late weaning will create unhealthy dependence, put the child in control, and generally contribute to a "spoiled child." Both experience and research have shown this not to be true. Studies comparing groups of babies who are identified as securely attached to the mothers with matched controls described as insecurely attached show that the securely attached babies (those who are not weaned before their time) actually grow to be more independent, separate more easily from their mothers, move into new relationships with more security and stability and are, in fact, easier to discipline.

Over the past ten years in our breastfeeding center we have studied our own patients who were not weaned before their time and noticed that these children are easier to discipline, show less anger, and undergo less anxiety in their transition from one developmental stage to another.

Even though you may feel secure with the pace at which you are weaning your child, be prepared for well-meaning advisors to shake your confidence a bit by exclaiming, "What? You're still nursing?" The subtle accusation here is that you are creating overdependency, that you are being possessive, that you are allowing your child to control you. Possessiveness means keeping a child from doing what he needs to do because of some need you have. This is unhealthy and not in accordance with the attachment style of parenting we teach throughout this book. But by nursing your child as long as he needs to nurse, you are meeting his needs and developing his trust in you. Have confidence in your mothering style and seek consultation from trusted, like-minded advisors. Natural weaning is a balance between the mother's willingness to release the baby and the baby's readiness to separate from the mother.

How to wean. There are two phases in weaning—detachment and substitution. As your baby is detached from the nourishment of your milk and solid food is substituted for it, other forms of emotional nourishment should be substituted for the emotional detachment from your breast. Here are some tips:

1. **Try to breastfeed your infant for nutrition for at least one year.** One year is a somewhat arbitrary figure, but it is in keeping with current medical teaching. In fact, most species of animals breastfeed their young until they triple their birthweight, which in human infants is around a year of age. Weaning begins between one and two years because the child is physically able to separate from mother (e.g., by walking). At the same time he develops an interest in maneuvering food with his hands, and the verbal ability to express his desires.

   At around one year the toddler reaches a milestone that aids him in weaning—the development of object permanence. During the first nine to twelve months, a baby does not yet have the memory skills to realize that mother exists when he cannot see her. Between one and two years a toddler can develop a mental picture of mother even when she is in another room; he, as it were, carries mother with him as he explores his environment. The cognitive ability facilitates weaning.

2. **Weaning should take place from person to person, not from person to thing.** As baby weans from mother's breast, another person should substitute other forms of nourishment, and this person naturally should be father.
3. **Wean gradually.** Weaning by desertion—leaving baby to go on a get-away holiday—is definitely to be avoided. Detachment not only from the mother's breast but from mother herself places unnecessary stress on a baby. The time-honored weaning method of "don't offer, don't refuse" seems to work the best for most mothers and babies. Between one and three years, as babies are naturally weaned into other relationships, they periodically return to mother as their home base for nutritional and emotional refueling.

   Be prepared for increases in nursing frequency as toddlers return to their secure home base during periods of high need or stress. Two-year-olds will often spend several months needing to nurse nearly as often as a newborn. While this will sometimes be perceived as a nuisance or an overdependency, it is a normal and healthy state of development as baby is returning to a known home base in order to be fulfilled with a relationship he knows and from which he develops a comfortable feeling that now it is okay to proceed into less-known relationships or more independent stages.
4. **Develop create alternatives to breastfeeding.** After your infant has been nursing for a year, this relation-

ship is so beautifully fixed in his developing mind that some toddlers give absolutely no indication of slowing down their nursing frequency. Many mothers have told us, "He waits for me to sit down and then pounces." The child's developing memory is like a big record; he cuts grooves in this record. The nursing groove is probably one of the deepest your child will ever cut, and he therefore returns to it frequently until other grooves are cut in his memory record.

The age at which children are willing to accept alternatives to breastfeeding is extremely variable. Expect nap nursing and night nursing to be the last feedings to go. Many toddlers retain a desire to breastfeed off to sleep well into the second and third year.

It is helpful to develop creative alternatives when your toddler is in need of comforting. If you only offer your breast as a solution, it will be harder for him to settle for anything else as he gets older. Toddlers may want to nurse when they are bored or need your attention, yet a story or a romp in the backyard may be even closer to what the child wants. Consider weaning a toddler as broadening your relationship, not a loss of a relationship. As with all parenting styles, there is a balance. Sometimes mothers do seem overattached to babies in that their total relationship revolves around breastfeeding. If you begin to feel that you are resenting so much breastfeeding, it is time to slow down and consider other ways of relating to your child. As you develop more playful interactions as alternatives to breastfeeding, your child will gradually learn to be content with them as a substitute.

Ideally it is the baby who weans from the mother. A gradual and timely weaning is a beautiful way for child and mother to cement their bond.

QUESTIONS AND ANSWERS

Q. Our three-month-old needs holding all the time and nurses frequently. I can't get any work done. Help!

Your baby is a baby for only a very short time. First define your priorities; housework should not be among them. As one mother shared with us, "I was a compulsive floor cleaner until I realized that the floor doesn't have feelings." You may have to temporarily lower your standards if you are a perfectionist. List the things that really bother you and must get done and limit your attention to those jobs, or ask your husband for help, or hire help. Wear your baby in a sling-type baby carrier. This allows you to "work and wear," enabling you to get things done around the house but also comfort your baby. Some babies are "in arms" infants for the first six months, then enjoy freestyle movements on the floor and sitting and playing awhile by themselves. Remember, you are getting something done by caring for your baby. You are doing the most important job in the world—raising a human being.

Q. I am prone to getting breast infections—over the past two months I have had four. My doctor thinks I may have to wean my baby but I don't want to. What am I doing wrong?

It is important to take inventory of what might be precipitating factors in these recurrent breast infections. Are you going too long between feedings? If you have an easy baby who sleeps a long time between feedings, your breasts may not be emptied enough and the residual milk may be inviting infection. Fatigue and stress are also common culprits. Are you getting enough rest? Are there major changes in your life, such as a move or a family trip? Beware of the "busy nest syndrome," which drains your energy.

An improperly fitting bra or underwire, pressure from the strap of a baby carrier or even unusual sleeping positions may create constriction of the breast. Some lactation consultants have reported that vigorous upper arm exercises, such as jumping rope, aerobics, or pushing a heavy lawn mower, may increase the risk of breast infections. Try your best to empty your breasts as much as possible with each feeding and as frequently as possible. If these suggestions are not working, seek consultation from a certified lactation consultant.

Q. What foods should I eat and which should I avoid while breastfeeding?

You should maintain the well-balanced diet that you had during your pregnancy. Avoid junk foods, which are high in calories and low in nutrition. Try to eat some of the four basic food groups every day. Even if you wish to hasten the return to your prepartum weight, avoid crash diets; they are not healthy for either mother or baby. Exercise is the safest way for the lactating mother to control her weight.

Most nursing mothers need at least 2,000 nutritious calories a day, plus at least eight glasses of water. As for what foods to avoid, some gas-producing foods which may or may not upset your baby are: raw cabbage, cauliflower, onions, broccoli, brussels sprouts, green peppers, and turnips. Caffeine-containing foods and drinks such as colas, chocolate, and coffee may upset the baby if taken in excess. Babies may also be allergic to the dairy products or even other foods in your diet, even if you show no signs of these allergies (see Key 17). Except for these foods, you can usually enjoy a normal diet during breastfeeding.

Q. I am a tense person. How can I relax better during nursing?

The way to create a relaxing atmosphere during breastfeeding is to develop a "nursing station." This is an area in your home that is especially set up for the nursing pair, with your favorite chair (preferably a rocking chair with arms at a comfortable height to support your arms while holding the baby), plenty of pillows, a footstool, soothing music, a relaxing book, nutritious nibbles, and lots of juice and water. Take the phone off the hook or have it next to you. This nursing station is like a nest within your home to which you can retreat with your baby, so you can more easily give him the quality and quantity of time that he needs.

If you have a toddler who still needs a lot of attention, set up your station on a pad or mattress on the floor with special time-out activities such as snacks, music, books, and special toys. This gives him access to you and reassures him that he is still important. Consider doing this in his room, where you can keep an eye on him. The hormone prolactin will naturally exert a relaxing effect on the breastfeeding mother. Nursing frequently keeps your prolactin levels high and increases the relaxing effect.

Q. How can my husband help in breastfeeding?

One father in a successful breastfeeding family summed it up very wisely, "I can't breastfeed our baby, but I can create an environment that helps my wife breastfeed better." Fathers can bathe with, walk with, play with, and help with baby—

changing, burping, and soothing, him. Breastfeeding is indeed a family affair.

Q. When will my milk come in?

Your true milk begins to appear between the second and fifth day after your baby's birth, depending on whether this is your first baby, the fatigue level of your birthing experience, how well the baby learns to latch on to your breasts, and how frequently and effectively the baby sucks. Until your true milk appears, baby is getting the "pre-milk" called colostrum, which is very rich in protein, immune factors and other ingredients beneficial to the newborn.

Q. If I have a low milk supply, will drinking more water help make more milk?

Studies have shown that drinking more fluids does not increase the milk supply; and if you force yourself to drink too much you can feel quite uncomfortable. If you are not drinking enough you will know it by concentrated urine and constipation. Breastfeeding causes most mothers to be thirstier than usual. If you "drink to thirst" and perhaps a glass extra, you should be fine.

Q. I've had a plugged duct for a week and the pain in my nipple is almost more than I can stand. There is a little white dot on my nipple that wasn't there before. How can I get rid of it?

The little white dot you see is just the "tip of the iceberg," or in this case the tip of a long strand of congested milk that is filling one of your milk ducts. If the standard remedies for unplugging the duct (warm soaks, massage, letting baby suck on the plugged side first at each feeding, and careful attention to perfect position and latch-on) are not working, you will have to get more vigorous in your approach. Have someone else apply firm pressure massage to your breast, starting at the chest wall and working down toward the nipple, using a goopy lubricant so the plugged duct can be worked out. This will be painful and may take a long time if the plug is a long one. You will actually see a strand of spaghettilike material extruding from the nipple pore, and eventually milk will flow freely again. If you catch this at the beginning, you can usually get the plug released by using a nursing position that employs gravity: place your baby on the bed and get on all fours so your breasts hang straight down, then let him suck strong and long.

GLOSSARY

Areola the dark area of the breast surrounding the nipple.
Breast shield a plastic cup with opening for the nipple, worn inside the bra. Used to draw out flat or inverted nipples for more successful breastfeeding.
Colostrum the first milk the baby receives after birth.
Foremilk the first, watery milk the baby receives at each feeding; it is low in fat and protein (see **hindmilk**).
Half-life the time required after ingestion of a drug for its concentration in the blood to be reduced by half.
Hindmilk the milk that the baby receives after 30 to 60 seconds or more of sucking; it is higher in fat and protein than the first milk or foremilk.
Immunoglobulins the germ-fighting substances present in breast milk.
Induced lactation starting the flow of breast milk in the absence of natural milk-producing hormones; used when an adoptive mother wishes to nurse.
Lactase an enzyme that helps in the digestion of lactose, or milk sugar.
Lactoferrin a special protein in breast milk that aids in the absorption of iron, protecting the baby against anemia.
Lactose natural milk sugar.
Letdown reflex see **milk ejection reflex**
Milk ejection reflex the outpouring of hindmilk from the milk glands into the milk sinuses, often signaled by a tingling sensation in the breasts.

Milk sinuses reservoirs where milk collects in the breast before being released to the nipple.

Oxytocin a hormone secreted by the pituitary gland and stimulated by suckling. Released shortly after birth, it hastens the return of the uterus to its normal size. During breastfeeding, oxytocin causes the tissue around the milk glands to contract and squeeze out milk.

Prolactin the "milk-producing" or "mothering" hormone, secreted by the pituitary gland and stimulated by suckling; it has a relaxing effect and heightens maternal instincts.

RESOURCES

- **Association for Breastfeeding Fashions,** P.O. Box 4378, Sunland, CA 91041.
- **La Leche League International,** PO Box 1209, Franklin Park, IL 60131-8209, 1-800-LA LECHE or (708) 455-7730.
- **Lactation Institute,** 16161 Ventura Blvd., Suite 223, Encino, CA 91436.
- **Medela Co.,** 1-800-435-8316. In Illinois, call collect (815) 455-6920.
- **Nojo Inc.,** 22942 Arroyo Vista, Rancho Santa Margarita, CA 92688, 1-800-541-5711.

INDEX